TO BE A PERSON

by

Jennifer Kate Olson

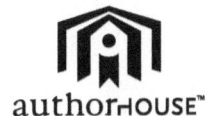

authorHOUSE™

1663 LIBERTY DRIVE, SUITE 200
BLOOMINGTON, INDIANA 47403
(800) 839-8640
WWW.AUTHORHOUSE.COM

First published by AuthorHouse 08/31/04

ISBN: 1-4184-9205-1 (sc)

Library of Congress Control Number: 2004096157

Printed in the United States of America
Bloomington, Indiana

This book is printed on acid-free paper.

I DEDICATE THIS BOOK TO:

Marie Moore and
Dr. Chris Frogley

Table of Contents

PREFACE ix

CHAPTER 1: THE BEGINNING OF MY JOURNEY............................. 1

CHAPTER 2: TRIALS AND TRIBULATIONS OF THERAPY............. 5

CHAPTER 3: THERAPY GETS SERIOUS 9

CHAPTER 4: SMITH-WARREN SCHOOL... 27

CHAPTER 5: MAIN STREAMING ME INTO
            PICKWICK SCHOOL.. 31

CHAPTER 6: EVANS JUNIOR HIGH SCHOOL 39

CHAPTER 7: OTTUMWA HIGH SCHOOL 45

CHAPTER 8: OTTUMWA HEIGHTS COLLEGE............................... 49

CHAPTER 9: THE IN BETWEEN EVENTS AND THOUGHTS
            OF THE FIRSTTWENTY YEARS OF MY LIFE 51

CHAPTER 10: LIFE GOES ON 55

CHAPTER 11: THE MIRACLES OF GOD... 59

CHAPTER 12: BITS AND PIECES FROM MY LIFE......................... 63

CHAPTER 13: THE HANDICAPPED ADULT GROUP...................... 69

CHAPTER 14: SPECIAL PEOPLE AND OTHER THINGS 73

CHAPTER 15: INDIAN HILLS COMMUNITY COLLEGE 79

CHAPTER 16: LIFE IN BURGE HALL AT
    THE UNIVERSITY OF IOWA 87

CHAPTER 17: SUMMER OF HELL....................................... 97

CHAPTER 18: OUR FIRST APARTMENT 103

CHAPTER 19: REST OF THE TIME AT
    THE UNIVERSITY OF IOWA 107

CHAPTER 19: SECOND AVENUE 111

CHAPTER 20: SHANNON DRIVE 115

CHAPTER 22: FIFTIETH BIRTHDAY PARTY................................ 119

EPILOGUE 121

PREFACE

We come into this world as innocent children,
And if we choose to do so, we leave as
   CHILDREN OF GOD.

                              Deb

This is a story of how I live with Cerebral Palsy (CP), a neuromuscular disease. I have all five types of CP which is very rare. The types that are more noticeable in me than others are: spastic, anthetoid, and athetosis. I also have to a small degree, very noticeable symptoms of the grimaces and convulsions (seizures) CP. I am classified as a walking quadriplegic with very little feeling from the breast line down. The degrees of CP can go from mild to severe and the symptoms can be brought on as a result of an injury or disease before or during birth or in early infancy.

I began writing this book in 1976 after many memories went through my mind over and over for a long period of time, which I felt was a sign from God. I had three purposes for the book when I first began writing. First, I wanted to share my life with others, this included the pains and joys that were part of me, and at the same time, I wanted to let people know that God never gives us more than we can handle. My second purpose was to demonstrate that the disabled actually do have a chance in life. Finally, I wanted to inspire other disabled people to fight for hopes and dreams and to let them know that they are not alone in their fight for survival.

I have shared my life in a variety of ways; through contributions from other people that have known me in some way, songs, poems, and prayers. I have acknowledged the authors of the works that are not mine. To protect everyone, all but my name is changed. At the time I started writing my book, I was fairly ambulatory but as I grew older, the effects of my CP deteriorated to the point that I am wheelchair dependent and I need help with many things on a daily basis.

I would like to start now by sharing a poem that deals with the aspect of life for disabled

individuals. The view is from a parent, but I feel that she is able to say a lot when it comes to someone living with a disability. I liked the poem very much when I first read it that I wanted to share the special meaning with others.

Mrs. Massimilla wrote this poem shortly after giving birth to a mentally handicapped son. She had the intentions of serving two purposes, which she did, in writing this poem. One, she was able to let go of some of the anger and hurt that she felt upon hearing that her son was one of chosen ones to be one of the many handicapped individuals in society. Second, through her poem, she helped many parents come to a deeper, clearer understanding of what it is like to have a handicapped child and to let other parents know that they were not alone. She wanted to say, "I know what you're going through, but if I can make it, you can too!"

HEAVEN' VERY SPECIAL CHILD

A meeting was held quite far from Earth "It's time again
for another birth."
Said the Angels to the Lord above "This child will need
much love."
His progress may seem very slow Accomplishments he
may never show.
And he'll require extra care from the folks he'll meet
down there.
He may not run or laugh or play his thoughts may seem
quite far away.
In many ways he won't adapt and he'll be known as
handicapped.
So let's be careful where he's sent we want his life to be
content.
Please Lord, find the parent who will do a special job for
you.
They will not realize right away the leading role they're
called to play.
But with this child sent from above comes stronger faith
and richer love.
And soon they'll know the privilege given In caring for
this gift from Heaven.
This precious child so meek and mild Is Heaven's Very
Special Child.

Edna Massimilla

So sit back and relax as you read, TO BE A PERSON!

CHAPTER 1: THE BEGINNING OF MY JOURNEY

I was born shortly after midnight on April 30, 1954. My parents were not emotionally ready to deal with a normal child, let alone dealing with a defective child, and therefore they had many problems in accepting me. Through this lack of coping with the situation as most parents learn to do, my parents showed strong evidence of an emotional instability disability. So in order for them to cope with my disability, I had to endure daily abuse along with the effects of my CP. The only reason that I was able to learn to move on my own was because I wanted to be able to escape some of the abuse.

Although my birth was a normal birth process, my head was born several moments before my body, which could therefore have caused some of the severe brain damage. The brain can live three minutes without oxygen before any real brain damage occurs. My brain was denied this crucially needed oxygen before my body was out of my mother's womb, which resulted in my having CP. The doctors finally had to break my collarbone in order to help my mother save me. CP is severe damage to the brain and motor system.

Little was known about CP the time. The doctor gave my father the chance to tell my mother that I had CP. But he didn't tell her! My mother was very ill at the time of my birth and father did not want to risk losing his wife by giving her the shocking news. I often wondered at times when I was living at home trying to cope with my disability and the abuse, if I would had been better off if they had let me die.

1

For a better understanding of CP and how it affects me, perhaps it would be helpful if I gave a definition of the condition. CP is a neuromuscular disease that involves a lesion of the brain which is chiefly characterized by spasms. Another name for CP is "Little's Disease." There are five types of CP, and it is possible for some victims to be mentally impaired. The types of spasms caused by this disability comes in the form of sudden/ temporary contractions of the muscles. These movements, which are part of my problem, can be a nuisance when I am busy working on simple everyday activities. Like when I am writing or trying to cut something, my food or a loose thread, or performing a simple daily activity such as getting dressed or eating.

In most cases the manifestations of CP mainly occur in early childhood and are present in varying degrees of paralysis, motor or limb involvement speech and hearing difficulties, mental retardation, and convulsions. Often the victim does not understand why this happened to him/her because they just want to be like other people. But it is also true that the people who have trouble accepting the disabled, can receive the same type of brain damage which may or may not result in getting CP or another disabling condition, if they are in a serious accident or are seriously ill for a long time. And for many this is a hard fact of life which they cannot accept!

In my case, the doctors knew that there was brain damage before the time of my birth. I was injured practically from the time of conception, but while mother carried me in her womb, more damage took place.

My daily problems include mobility, walking (I have trouble walking straight), using my hands, (I have problems with spastic movements in my hands and arms at times when I do simple every day activities), speech (my speech is difficult at times for others to understand and my face will make facial grimaces while I am talking), and coordination. The general public has often thought of me as an alcoholic because of my inabilities in doing simple things such as walking or talking. When eating or drinking, many have told me that I remind them of a "drunkard." Believe me, if this comes from someone you think you are close to, it hurts.!

During the first few weeks of my life I was in the hospital. Most of this time I was in an incubator, a machine with a lot of tubes to supply medicine and oxygen to the baby. The oxygen that was given to me was the only way that I could breathe. During the time that I was there, it was necessary for everyone and everything to be sterilized before making any type of contact with me. The incubator was considered as a life support and monitor for me. The doctors were not sure if I would live because my heart had stopped several times. The incubator had been the beginning of the long medical help that my life would require.

After my coming out of the incubator (which I was in for twenty - eight days), I can imagine the happy feeling that my mother or any other mother would have when she was able to hold her baby for the first time since birth. Unfortunately, my mother did not feel this way. It was necessary for mother to have surgery immediately after giving me life, so she didn't know for three days that I was deformed. It was hard for her to accept me because she thought that she had given birth to a "normal" baby. Today, the separation of mother and child isn't so long and there is more support given to a mother in a similar situation. Today, it has also been shown that without maternal bonding in similar circumstances, the child suffers more physical and emotional abuse.

There were to be many trips to our local doctor and to Iowa City. But, in the beginning, I thought that my parents didn't mind. I would find out a lot different in years to come. Once money and health problems arose, the trips to Iowa City had to be stopped. I had became a target for physical abuse. Mother's rejection of a disabled child was something she felt ashamed of. (For many years, I felt I owed them a lot for everything that they "tried" to do for me. But I finally realized that most of the progress that I made was through my own determination and God's help.)

Although I came into this world in the early hours of the morning, I feel that I still knew that God had a special assignment for me to do. My assignment was/is to try to make this time on Earth a little more easier and accessible for the disabled. Thus, my reasoning for feeling that God wanted me to write this book to help other disabled individuals and their families to learn to cope with the situation.

HANDICAPPED

Hands that shake.
Arms laying limp.
Needs for assistance.
Drugs for helping you.
Ideas for the future.
Caring for each other.
Achievements to be made.
Pain that never goes away.
Patience is an important key.
Education to be pursued.
Dreams that never come true.

Deb

Author's Note: These feelings, emotions, and ideas are virtually needed in everyday living in order to survive.

CHAPTER 2: TRIALS AND TRIBULATIONS OF THERAPY

I was between one and two when the effects of my handicap was first totally realized. The future was unclear, but I could win the fight to survive daily living in the years to come if my family and I would do the hard work and if I could concentrate with my determination to keep the progress coming.

When I was between the ages of two and four, Dr. Tutor and Dr. Slater, the doctors who had evaluated me at the Children's Hospital School in Iowa City, held a conference with my family. It was decided from the results of many tests and evaluations that had been done on me, that through a lot of hard work I had a chance. This news came as a blessing considering I had not seen any chance to move as of yet. I would have to learn to make adjustments and adaptions to meet my needs, but I could do it. At first this was very hard to believe, but I wanted to give myself a fighting chance.

As the time went by, my family realized that we would need help in paying for the trips to Iowa City. In the beginning, it was necessary for me to make this trip every month, then it became every three months, and the time span ended up as being every six months. If I had not missed so many appointments, I would probably still be going there today. A lot of money was needed to pay for my braces, diagnostic testing, and anything else that the doctors felt that I would benefit from. In our time of need, my family was informed about a government program called Clinical Pay.

This program agrees to pay for everything except the registration fee in Iowa City for those that qualify for this type of assistance. It was very hard for me to get accepted into this program.

Had it not been for Rhonda Little, who was a Public Health Nurse at the time, I most likely would not had been able to receive assistance from this program. It was on one of Mrs. Little's visits with my family that she was told about our difficulties in getting assistance from the Clinical Pay Program. After Mrs. Little spoke with the program representative at the Court House, it was determined I was eligible for assistance from the program. But my parents still refused to keep the appointments. They acted like it was wasting their "precious" time in taking me somewhere to get help so that I would be able to move and do things on my own for awhile.

Looking back, I felt sorry for them until recently when I found out from one of the doctors that they released me in order to keep my family quiet and not harassing them all of the time. What my family did not or does not realize is that I am the one who suffers from the consequences, not them!

The progress would go from not being able to move at all, to moving around like the average person, to the present condition of being limited to a certain amount of mobility. Therapy would cause many heart breaking moments. But in the end, visible progress would be made. Not only was I not able to talk or move my limbs, I was a quadriplegic.

After it was first noticed that I did not have the ability to move on my own, which was very frustrating for me, a series of home exercises and patterning was started. Patterning was physically painless but necessary for any type of progress to be made. The first step in patterning was to move my legs back and forth in a crawling manner. How many people have this process done to them in order to move? The answer isn't important. What is important is that I needed to go through it in order for me to start becoming independent. Body rubs and moving the rest of my body in a mannerly fashion were also included in this program.

I was totally confused on the first day that these treatments began because I had not seen any other family member having to go through this type of program, or any other program for that matter. This program took many, many months before any type of movement was noticed. Eventually however, all of the hard work paid off when I began moving my limbs by myself. All of these treatments began in Iowa City and continued through the years that I was in therapy.

For many weeks, months, and yes, years, there was not any noticeable changes. Just slow progression requiring much patience on everyone's part. Gradually, I was able to see my body move. This type of therapy was continued at home until I started going to the Smith-Warren School for the physically disabled for treatment. I began my treatments in 1958 at this school.

Each day would begin by Miss Hendrix, my occupational therapist, going through my home exercises, patterning, expanding my lungs by rubbing ice on them, rubbing my entire body to stimulate movements in my limbs, and stretching my fingers so that I could use them. Most of the time when my hands are not being used, I either keep them in a fist or half way closed, or I will sit on them so that they will not shake so much. However, using these methods do not and can not always stop the spastic movements in my hands.

After Miss Hendrix finished with me, Mr. Jarvis, and Mrs. Dean took turns in working with me. Mr. Jarvis would work with my entire body, but mainly on my legs. Mrs. Dean worked with me so that I could learn to talk.

Later in my life, I had the chance to visit with these people about working with me. They all said there was very little hope for me at first. But the longer they worked with me, the better things started to look. They were all very proud of me and the accomplishments that I made for myself.

Jennifer Kate Olson

THE DREAM

I had a dream I could walk.
    And yes, I could even talk.
My hands no longer shook.
    Now people had no reason to look.
I dreamed that I could see.
    How to be happy and free.
I dreamed I could hear.
    No longer would people sneer.
Oh, if only this was true.
    Then I'd be just like you.
But no longer am I in despair.
    For I'll find my place somewhere.
But then I awoke.
    And listened to the words I had spoke.
Unlike the birds flying high and free.
    I knew it wouldn't ever happen to me.

Deb

Author's Note: Although I can still do most of these things without any problems, I still have a few difficult moments. But with a lot of patience, determination, and self confidence, I eventually get everything done. In 1998, it became medically necessary for me to limit my walking and become more dependent on my wheelchairs (I have both the electric and manual type). It is now 2003 and I am totally dependent on my wheelchairs.

CHAPTER 3: THERAPY GETS SERIOUS

CP affects the way I use to where performing simple everyday tasks is very difficult for me to do. Imagine what it is like to have a fight everyday just to get dressed or eat a meal. I want to scream because I can't do things the way I want to, and that is so frustrating that it hurts.

Second, my speech is impaired so other people have trouble understanding me. This is especially true with "L" words and it is sometimes hard for me to pronounce names. Words like "lucky" and "liberal" come out sounding garbled and distorted. Last names are particularly difficult for me to pronounce and I periodically refer to my teachers by their first name. No matter how hard I try some people just can't carry a conversation with me. At times that really hurts me!

Finally, my legs are affected and I cannot walk as well as most people. Often when strangers hear me talk or see me out walking they think that I am drunk. But I am not drunk because I can not drink. I have only had one drink in my life, and that drink set me back so far that I do not want another one!

I was given therapy to teach me how to move. First, I was in occupational therapy, so that I could learn to use my hands. I began my lessons by performing simple everyday tasks such as dressing and feeding myself. Then as I grew older, I tried to work long and hard on other activities involving the use of my hands such as typing and weaving. If my progress did not please my family, I would endure more emotional, physical, verbal, and sexual abuse (which no one knew that I was having done to me.) It was not enough to see me struggle to do everyday activities, but I had to endure the pain of abuse too!

I had many therapist that would work with me here but it was Miss Hendrix who worked with me the most. In fact, I feel that she was the best therapist that I had because throughout the years of working together, we seemed to come closer together. Miss Hendrix was no stranger to me because she and her family were among the many people that came to our house to work with me doing the home exercises and both families were close friends and her Dad was our doctor. Miss Hendrix was a caring person and was deeply concerned about every student whom she worked with.

In the occupational therapy room I worked very hard on coordination to learn to stabilize my hands and arms. In fact, this was part of the process that was necessary in order to dress and feed myself. I wonder how many people have to stop and think about these problems before doing them. For the physically handicapped, it DOES present some problems. I will try to explain this to you the best way I can.

When buying my clothes, people would look for slacks with stretch bands and pull over tops. This made dressing easier, if much less fashionable. Also, I did not experience as much frustration, and this is still true today as well. (Although I am an adult now, I still have trouble getting dressed at times. Dressing not only requires good hands, but it also involves a lot of hard work and concentration. On some days it is a battle just getting dressed for the day; and at times, I wonder if the frustration is worth it.)

Learning to dress myself was to take three hard years in my life, but I always would/will have some problems. When I have to button something, I just say, "it's time to have a fight with the buttons fight."

The task of dressing was part of everyday life that I had to learn fast in order to put my clothes and braces on by myself. Namely, my worst problem was getting my hands to stay still while I was putting my braces on. I was very much more spastic when I was younger and it was a job at times to get my hands to open up to tie my shoe laces or buckle the buckles on my braces, let alone getting completely dressed by myself.

First, I would have many days that were frustrating because I could not do anything. Days when simply pulling my clothes on would be hard because the spastic movements were too severe; I really felt out of place on these days and I still do at certain times today. Then I would/do have a few days where I could/can dress myself most of the way without any help. Finally, there would be days known to be triumphant because absolutely no help was needed; on these days I felt like I would win the battle. Then I would get discouraged the next day because the battle would start all over.

I remember that Miss Hendrix had a lot of patience when working with me. She would sit in front of me holding a board shaped like a man. On one side the man had two shirts on it. The first shirt had buttons on it and the second shirt had snaps on it. Miss Hendrix would have me work on this board man to master these skills before practicing with my own clothes. On the other side of this man were two layers of buckles and zippers that met me daily. Here again, I practiced these skills on a board before doing it with my own clothes. So that I could practice tying laces a wooden shoe was used. (Nevertheless zipping, tying, buttoning a man made of wood and doing the same to myself were two different matters altogether.) This also meant that I needed assistance until these skills were mastered. To many, this may seem very elementary, but for me, it was an IMPORTANT step for me to be able to function in life. At the time I was learning to forever fight buckles and shoe laces, there wasn't anything with velcro fastening. This was unfortunate because velcro made things easier for everyone. Dressing would never be easy for me because coordination and spastic movements would always be a problem, velcro or no.

Eating was a whole new arena of problems for me. First, there was special dishes I used until I was able to get more stability to use regular dishes, or as much as I ever would have. For instance, I would use a plate with suction cups on it to prevent the plate from moving around on me; also, I would use a built up fork or spoon until I was able to learn how to use regular utensils (however, I mainly use a tablespoon to make eating easier.) Because the fork and spoon was hard to find, Miss Hendrix would accommodate the regular utensils by taping a lot of foam rubber on the handles so that the silverware would meet my needs. These adapted utensils came in very handy when Smith-Warren would receive hot lunches for the students. While Smith-Warren was still behind the fire station, we received hot lunches from the Washington Junior High School. By using these utensils, I was able to feed myself without very much help or embarrassment. But after awhile, these utensils did not help me any more; however I used these utensils until Smith-Warren moved out on Williams Street, then I took my lunch.

Another aid that I used, and still use today, was a straw or a cup with handles on both sides of it until I became able to use a standard cup. Today the way that I hold my cup in my hands reminds people of a "drunkard." I really try to do my best! I always have had trouble holding a cup, I can do it but not the way other people do. Most people hold a cup with one hand, whereas I hold a solid side in my right hand and use my left hand to hold the bottom; this makes the cup more stable for me. When I am eating out, I will use a straw so that I will not embarrass anyone by the way that I hold my cup. Using a straw is much easier for me in the long run.

Other difficulties that I have in the area of eating includes cutting my food and making a mess. A great deal of coordination and stability is required in order for me to cut something up and/or out. First, one must have two "good" hands in order to cut something. I can do this but it is not very easy. Sometime when you have the opportunity, watch a five or six year old attempting to cut a piece of meat, add to it that the child is extremely cold or nervous, or in a hurry therefor shaking and clumsy, and you have a picture of what it is like for me as an adult to eat (I use that word loosely) a meal at any time in my life.

A second aspect in cutting is that one needs for his/her hands to be steady. Due to my spastic movements, there is always the possibility that the dishes or papers will move around while I am in the process of cutting. But as the old saying goes, "that's the way the ball bounces" or "the tomatoes" or "the peas" or "the eggs" or "the potatoes" or "anything else." Up through my early teens, I had, and still do, trouble eating neatly. By using the words "making a mess" I mean not only getting food all over me, but the floor and table too.

While at Smith-Warren, if I did not eat neatly, the next day I would have to watch myself eat in front of a mirror; when I did this, I usually would sit in the occupational therapy room which is very dramatic for a handicapped person. Believe me, I know! A table with a circle cut out of the center on one side was always in front of a mirror. At this table I was able to set right up to my plate so that there was no room for food to go anywhere but my mouth. It would depend on how bad of a mess that I made on the number of days that I had to do this. For instance, if I made a small mess, one or two days; but if it was a big mess, I was found to endure five to seven days of this. The reason behind this was believed to be if I watched myself making a mess, I would eat neater. No matter how hard I tried, this was not always the case though. I usually could not control jell - o which would end up in my lap or on the floor, or vegetables which would soar out of control in every direction. Occasionally, I even had trouble handling bread or milk.

I never thought about it until later in my life, but it now seems as if this was a type of punishment to make me feel guilty for being different. Many people ask me how my therapists got away with this. My reply: Easy! Because this was considered part of my treatments. But, I have carried this lesson in my heart all through my life. Every time I go out to eat, it still bothers me. At one restaurant in Ottumwa, Pearl's, the owners and waitress try to get me to relax and not worry if I make a mess. If I order a sandwich on the night they have an entree that I like Pearl comes out to see why, but deep down she always knows the answer.

"Sweetie don't worry about it, we can clean it up," she says. "Besides you usually don't make that much of a mess." I tell her that I know but it bothers me when I do.

"Well it shouldn't," Pearl says.

A number of people like Pearl, Harry, and Sylvia try to get me to relax about the way I eat; but I just can't. I guess that I still remember the days when I had to do my eating in front of a mirror, feeling humiliated watching myself mess myself, and hating myself more and more each time. I still criticize myself when I make a mess while eating.

Other activities and games were included in my treatments. I did exercises such as writing, putting beads and puzzles together, placing pegs into pegboards, and weaving. All of these activities were important in obtaining good coordination. In later years of therapy, I was taught to type to relieve the tension that I go through when I am trying to write.

I made things like rugs, place mats, potholders, and many other items. As I became older, these activities were to become a hobby and pastime. Whenever I had many of these craft items made, I would sell them for a little extra spending money for my family.

The games that we played, checkers and dominoes, perhaps had a therapeutic value as well as being a time when Miss Hendrix and I would feel like we could laugh together and tease each other as we went along. I remember one afternoon when we were playing dominoes and we were having a really good time; I ended up beating Miss Hendrix in the game, but I knew it was getting time for me to get back into the relaxation chair, a specially designed contraption which when tilted back was supposedly would make its occupant more relaxed and less spastic. It was very ironic that this chair was named so since I hated this chair very much. It reminded me of a high chair except this chair was much bigger and was on a platform with wheels. If I was in this chair at meal time, and I was tilted back because of being too spastic someone would have to feed me; which made me hate the chair all the more, and at the same time, made me think of it more as a high chair!

If I had to use one of these today, I don't think that I would have as many friends as I do now. That's how bad I hated this chair, and I don't think that my friends would have been able to accept this chair anymore than I could. As I said earlier, the purpose of this chair was supposedly to relax me by tipping me back. Depending on the degree of my spastic movements, the chair might be tipped back only slightly or at a ninety to a hundred and eighty degree angle. Nevertheless, whatever the angle it was a very odious ordeal for me.

On this particular afternoon when we were finished, Miss Hendrix said, "Debbie, I'm sorry but its time for you to get back into the relaxation chair."

"Do I have to?" I asked.

"Yes" she said.

I really dreaded this chair because I couldn't do anything by myself while in it. I was so relaxed on this particular afternoon that I pleaded with Miss Hendrix not to put me back in.

"I'll tell you what Debbie, I won't tilt you back as far as I usually do" was Miss Hendrix's reply.

Reluctantly, I told her "okay" and was strapped in for the rest of the day.

As the weeks went by, I began to get to the point where I could not unwind as much as I had and this worried Miss Hendrix very much. One afternoon the two of us talked about it. At this time no one knew about the daily abuse that I endured besides the problems from my handicap (and no one really did find out until I started main streaming into the regular school system.)

"Debbie, why is it that you don't seem to enjoy the games anymore?"

With some reluctance I said, "Why should I? I just have to go back into the chair anyway."

"Is that what's really bothering you?" (I was too scared to tell her the effects from the abuse was what was really bothering me.)

"Yes."

"But why Debbie?"

"I just feel like I'm trapped when I sit in the relaxation chair. I can't do anything without someone helping me."

"This is true, but we're only having you do it because I think it will help you Debbie. Do you understand?"

"Yes."

"Can I see you smile Debbie?"

"Yes." I gave her a fake smile but I was frowning on the inside though.

The lesson about fear was the most valuable one that I learned during the time Miss Hendrix was my therapist, and one I won't ever forget. We were doing stencil painting at the time I became afraid of Miss Hendrix, which was unusual at this time if I trusted someone. The stencil painting was brought in by Mrs. Walker, who was a mother of one of the students, and given to Miss Hendrix for the occupational students to do. Miss Hendrix showed me how to do this one day and then she had to leave the room for awhile. As I was painting my brush went dry, or so I thought, so I got up to wet it like I had seen Miss Hendrix do. Unfortunately, I got the brush too wet and it was still very wet when Miss Hendrix returned.

"Debbie did you wet this brush yourself?"

In a state of panic and fear, I told her "No."

"Are you sure about this Debbie?"

"Yes."

Miss Hendrix put my stencil painting away for a few days and talked to me about it again.

"Debbie are you sure you didn't wet this brush yourself? It's still very wet."

Although I was still very afraid, I confessed to her that I did wet the brush myself.

"Why did you lie to me?"

"I was afraid that you would be mad and hurt me." (By now I was use to being hurt whenever

I did something wrong.)

Her eyes widened, smile faded, and in a lower softer voice, she replied, "I don't understand

Debbie, I can't ever remember hurting you.'"

I told her that I didn't know what made me feel like this, but in reality it was an after fact of the abuse which made me feel this way, but I just panicked and became suddenly afraid of her.

"I'm going to ask Mr. Jarvis, the physical therapist and principal, to join us to talk about this."

The three of us talked for a very long time but I could not tell them why I was really afraid. I took my punishment, which was a spanking, and then Mr. Jarvis left the room. My parents were called after we talked and when I got home that night, I was punished more severely. When I came to school with some bruises the next day Miss Hendrix (who was beginning to suspect the abuse) asked me what happened. I told her that I fell so that I wouldn't have to tell her about the abuse. I was still scared and didn't think anyone would believe me if I did say something. Later in my life, my therapists found out there was abuse going on, and they tried to help me get out of the situation, but they were unsuccessful in doing so.

Miss Hendrix waited till the day after she, Mr. Jarvis and I talked then she said, "Debbie, I would not had been mad or hurt you in any way if you had told me the truth. I want to help you not hurt you. Do you understand?"

"Yes, it's just for some reason I got afraid. I don't know why. I am sorry for what I did." Little did Miss Hendrix know that I was punished at home for two months for this incident.

"Debbie, you know you can't do anymore stencil painting don't you?"

"Yes."

"You can go now and think about what I said."

"Debbie?"

"Yes?"

"Remember that I won't hurt you."

"I will."

A few days after this incident Miss Hendrix and I had another heart to heart talk. She explained to me that she had been working with me ever since my treatments began. "I remember Debbie at first there was so little hope. You were very badly injured from your handicap and it was very doubtful that you would make any progress. Your motivation, determination, and perseverance made up for your lack of movement. I am very close to you kids and I have a deep love for each of you." I told her that I could see now and I did not think I would ever be afraid again.

Unfortunately, I never got over my feelings of fear, which I think is natural for anyone that has been abused. I would/do go through daily life and still be very much afraid. Again, I think that this stems from the abuse I had to endure daily. I hope that Miss Hendrix or anyone else that has/ does know me, does not feel that they were wasting their time on me. Maybe some day all of my fears will go away, but until then, I will just have to live with them.

Other memories of Miss Hendrix include the days that she walked over to Pickwick (my elementary school for grades 3 - 6, after I began main streaming in my second year of third grade) and the years that I was in Girl Scouts.

While I was in Girl Scouts, Miss Hendrix tried to buy cookies from as many of the girls as she could. One year she came to the house to pick up her cookies. That night her suspicions about the abuse was verified; although the money for the cookies went to the Girl Scout office, she made the check out to me and taught me how to sign it before turning it in, she wanted to be sure she taught me how to do this for my adult life. During this lesson she was told not to bother because I was too dumb to understand. She had seen me with a lot of bruises, and she had just heard verbal and emotional abuse.

When I got to school the next day, she told me I would be going to her house instead of home. I pleaded with her not to get hurt or in trouble because of what she saw and heard the night before; she told me that she could protect us both. True to my fears, father was at her house causing trouble that night, I went home that night mainly to protect her and her family. The next day she and her father met me as the cab let me out so they could examine me. Again, I pleaded for them to stay safe. That night I was taken to my grandparents on my dad's side, but they would not let my parents have me. However, the next day my grandparents gave in and the abuse became more intense. Later in my life, both of my parents acknowledged and apologized for the abuse before they died.

As for walking over to Pickwick with me, most of the time she did this voluntarily. I remember the time that a large bulldog met us as we were getting off the bus. (Although I was going to Pickwick, I still rode the Smith-Warren school bus in the morning.) I hope that Miss Hendrix knew that I really appreciated her moral support.

These are just a few ways that professional people work with the handicapped, not only physically, but mentally and emotionally too. In working with the handicapped it is vitally important to give them moral support. It is from this support that one can find the means for fighting for his//her dreams. I feel that because I was given moral support, I was able to get the inner courage that was needed for me to succeed as much as possible.

The following paragraphs are from Miss Hendrix. When I wrote to her, she told me that it was very hard for her to remember very much because it has been a long time since we have seen each other or worked together. And she has worked with so many since then.

"I remember that Debbie had a number of problems performing daily activities due to a lack of co-contraction of muscles for joint stabilization."(This means because I was spastic, it took my brain longer to send a message to my arms and legs to perform a task.) "At the time I worked with Debbie, I had not had the advanced course of neural development treatment which places emphasis on the facilitation of movement after joint compression and joint stabilization. However, my observations of her movement patterns, when stabilized, provided the proper assessment of having her try to stabilize her arms while using her hands."

17

"Debbie worked long and hard to accomplish buttoning, lacing, and bow tying. Her independence was very important to her. Meal time was hard due to problems of head control, swallowing, and involuntary movements of arms and hands. One method that seemed to help was to have her steady her elbow on the table before dipping for food with the spoon or fork and taking it to her mouth. But because it was considered poor manners to eat with your elbow on the table, it took some strong convincing before Debbie would do this, but she finally realized that she made less of a mess and had more stability." (Another method was to hold my arms against my body, this seemed to help me at times.)

"Debbie always wanted to try doing activities that she saw her mother and older sister doing at home. She enjoyed the group homemaking activities." (I especially enjoyed the cooking we did.)

"One time she was so intent on making cookies, but because she was drooling, I threw her cookie dough away." (At first I was a little confused and hurt when Miss Hendrix did this, but after we talked it over, I understood her reasons. The second time I really concentrated on swallowing and staying dry on the chin. The cookies were delicious.)

During the time that the group was cooking, it seemed as if Miss Hendrix was only a step away. She was always willing to help any of us in any way that we needed her. I felt that Miss Hendrix knew how most of us felt as well as being a good therapist. During these times (early 50's through late 60's) she too had to fight society because she was a Negro. But I did not have any reservations about being with her, because in her own special way, Miss Hendrix was helping me open a new door for myself. Because Miss Hendrix was so near to me when working with me, I feel that this was part of her way of caring about me, and at the same time, showing me a way to do things so that I would have the opportunity to live independently.

"Another time Debbie insisted that I teach her how to knit because her mother was crocheting at home. Needless to say, teaching a seven year old girl with athetosis and spastic movements was probably one of the greatest challenges I have had as an occupational therapist. We finally had to substitute a knitting-rake for needles and Debbie made a knitted cap. Her determination was a strong balance for her lack of coordination. " (I wanted to be able to do everything a normal person could do.) "Debbie required very few adaptions but I did start her to use (for awhile) a built-up fork, spoon, and a built-up pencil holder. This made handling these objects easier."

"Most of the activities were chosen to improve bilateral coordination. Stringing beads was preliminary to lacing shoes as an example. I cannot remember all of the specific activities because

Debbie was always wanting to try activities that would be intellectually stimulating." (Although I was/am handicapped, the IQ tests verified me as being above average intellectually.) "It was always challenging to find activities that were suitable for both her movement level and her intellectual level."

"It was important to work with all of the other staff members (teacher, speech therapist, physical therapist, and Debbie's parents) so that her total program would meet her total needs. As she became older, it was important to help her develop the skills that would help her in attending a regular school program and have less concentration on therapy." (Deep down I feel that my being able to attend a regular school was to be a part of my program no matter what happened.)

As I went through the years of occupational therapy, each new therapist would try new and different methods of working with me. Each new method would provide a new experience for me. I was ready to learn what I could when I could. I remember working with Miss Lane who was fresh out of college when she worked with me. Most of her methods was more suitable for the younger students. One of the methods that she used was to have me lay down to relax before I started my treatments. Because she was used to working with younger students, she would sing lullabies in this time. This was very embarrassing for me because I was a teenager when she worked with me. I felt very sorry for her because she did not know how to work with me.

My next therapist was Mrs. Early. Because she was not sure of the future for me because of my limited movement ability, she was not sure how to work with me. During the first few years that Mrs. Early worked with me, she taught me how to type on an electric typewriter with a key guard on it. This knowledge was to be very valuable to me in my later years. In ninth grade, it was decided to send me to Iowa City to see how they felt about me attending our local high school, which had a lot of steps for me to climb up and down. It was Mrs. Early who performed the basic movement tests that had to be sent to Iowa City before I went up for my evaluation. Some of these tests were so elementary that we both felt out of place.

The following ideas are from Mr. Jarvis (a very kind and capable man it seemed to me then) that worked with me all the time I was in Physical Therapy. Physical Therapy was the second therapy session that I attended on a daily basis. This therapy was to work with my legs and strengthen my muscles. The work here is what helped me so that I could eventually stand and walk. I would begin each session by walking through parallel bars. At first, it was necessary for Mr. Jarvis to put me in position, but eventually I became able to do this by myself. Also, for awhile Mr. Jarvis would meet me at the end to turn me around. The parallel bars was how I became able to walk and stand to the best of my ability today. Steps were/ are a problem for me, both up and down.

"Debbie's physical therapy program began at Smith-Warren on March 16, 1958. Although I did not continue seeing her on a daily basis for therapy after she entered into a regular school program, I continued seeing Debbie until May 26, 1969. With Debbie wearing braces, it was necessary for me to set up an intensive exercise program. "

Next we moved over to the exercise table to work on strengthening my legs and muscles. I would do such things as sit-ups, leg rolls, and toe raisers. All of these were necessary in order for me to gain mobility and put my hip sockets back in place. At the time of my birth, my sockets were not properly in place. When Smith-Warren moved out on Williams Street, I would do many of these exercises in the swimming pool; I could not use the pool after starting over at Pickwick School because there was not enough time.

Since I had/have a problem walking, it was necessary for me to wear leg braces until the early part of 1963. In 1990, I wore half braces on my legs for awhile, but they did not seem to help so I discontinued wearing them. I had trouble convincing them that wearing braces for awhile was a part of the process for CP victims; maybe some day they will realize that I knew what I was talking about. Walking concerning steps and long distances would always cause problems for me; the more I walk the less strength that I have for other activities. Usually if I know that a long distance or steps were part of a field trip or planned activity, I would not go. Now I have a manual wheelchair to take with me on such trips. I also have an electric wheelchair that I used on Campus when I was attending the University of Iowa, work, and/or personal/necessary errands.

Some other equipment that I would use until I became able to walk included weights, I used these on different parts of my body at times; parallel bars, steps and a number of small articles, such as a ball, to work on my coordination. The ball was usually made of foam rubber or a soft baseball. The purpose of these items were to strengthen my muscles and improve my coordination so that I did not shake all the time. All of this equipment and small articles were included with my braces during the first few years of my life.

Due to the fact that hip sockets were out of place at birth, it was necessary to participate in a program called home exercises. A common name for these exercises was patterning. Patterning which was performed many times, was not painful but necessary. This was to work on my knees and hips so that I could walk. Mr. Jarvis, along with many other people that would help with the patterning, as well as myself, would work on bending my knees to encourage me to pick up my feet and use the heel-toe method of walking instead of walking on my tip toes. This was combined with rolling my legs in and out to get my hip sockets in place without having surgery. Because no one knew if this was possible, it was very hard for everyone to work on this step. Fortunately, through everyone's work, I was able to get them in place.

Another set of exercises was used to make progress and to gain gait control. I did these to eliminate the "little drunken soldier" look. These exercises was done on an exercise table or bike. Due to my spastic movements, it was necessary for me to learn how to keep my arms down and walk straight. It is sometimes hard for me to walk straight because my legs tend to scissor and get tangled up. When this happens too much, I am more liable to fall.

By using braces, I was taught how to keep my balance, so after I got out of braces, it was necessary for me to learn to keep my balance without anyone or anything helping me. Today, I either use a walker or hold on to someone's arm or shoulder to keep my balance if I feel unsteady or if I am trying to walk; but as of 2002, I am not allowed to walk anymore.

I had to learn all over what I had learned to do with my braces. I was frightened at times, but I kept my determination up so that I could become independent. One of the things I would do to get my balance was practice standing on one foot. First, I would do this in between the parallel bars until I got enough courage and strength to do it by myself. Then, I would stand on one foot in front of a mirror to see how I should look when my body was balanced. This activity would remind a non-handicapped person of playing hopscotch or jumping a rope. I also on strengthening my abdominal muscles, dorsi flexor, and learned how to use my right side more than my left side. For a long time I used my left side just as much as my right side. Now I sometimes use my right hand to stabilize my left hand. Today I use both hands an equal amount. While doing all of these therapeutic activities, I eventually became able to do most everyday activities.

After taking a fifteen minute break, I would go to my last therapy session for the morning, which was Speech and Hearing. Here one would find students being taught how to talk and going through periodic hearing tests. Picture in your mind if you can, a child between the ages of five and nine saying his/her first words or hearing a sound through a hearing aid for the first time, then you get a general idea of what this therapy accomplishes. Most people are able to begin talking, or at least communicate intelligently, by the age of two; but for many handicapped people, they can only talk through muttered sounds or by pointing to what they want. Mrs. Dean would work with me so that I could talk instead of just making sounds.

The best part of this therapy is when you get to hear yourself talk for the first time in your life.

But with the good, comes the pain of knowing that not everyone will be able to understand you.

That is why today most students are given therapy right in the classroom so that their fellow classmates can go through each step with them. I think that this is good because people get the chance to see the pain and frustration that a handicapped person goes through just to be able to talk and hear.

Speech and Hearing involved many activities for me. I was taught how to use my mouth and tongue to form words, even how to take a sound and make it into a word. This is a process everyone must go through, but for me, it took years and years again. Here again, I had many different therapist, but it was Mrs. Dean who worked with me the longest. Mrs. Dean was more experienced than any of the other therapist I worked with. Unlike Mr. Jarvis, who I only worked with for a hour each day, Mrs. Dean and I became close of the two hours per day that we spent together so that I could talk.

Other therapists, I cannot remember how many, would try some of the newer methods on me. One method that they would have me use when a person had a tone of voice that I could not hear, was to try to follow their lips so that I would not have many problems. But with many, this was and still is, impossible to do because people move around too much. Nevertheless, I have learned to get by the best I can. I would do such exercises as practicing in front of a mirror saying "l" words and saying some of the everyday words like "apple, car or house." Mrs. Dean would use word cards with pictures on them and have me watch her lips as she said the words; very much like teaching a toddler to talk, only I was about four years old and my tongue didn't want to cooperate and/or work with me. It is still very hard for me to say "l" words along with other sounds. Mrs. Dean had me keep a notebook with all their words and meanings that I worked long and hard to say. However, in my younger years she would have to do this task because I couldn't do it myself.

Another exercise was to have me read out loud so that I could learn to speak more clearly. I read from my texts, magazines with related study materials, or the weekly readers that we received. This also helped in my studying. Because most of my time at school was consumed with therapy, my uncle Harley, who was a teacher in the regular school system, helped me with my scholastic studies to keep me up with my age level. I also read prayers out of a book when it was my turn to give the prayer. By reading out loud, I was able to learn how I sounded to other people. I can't really describe it but to say it sounds awful!

Hearing was also part of this therapy. I would go through periodic hearing tests because I had/have hearing problems. These tests would go from very low to very high tones and many of these tones were/are a problem for me. When I was going to school I would sit close to the front so that I could read peoples' lips. Now I sometimes use hearing aids so that I can hear better; I have a forty to ninety-five percent hearing loss.

Therapy was an important part of my life. I went through many trying moments which taught me to keep everything inside, which was not to be the case in later years. As I went through the years of therapy, I was told in order to be accepted by society I would have to keep my feelings inside. I have carried this lesson in my heart all my life, and when things become too much for me, I go through a period of depression. Like many other handicapped individuals I try not to let things get the best of me, but it does not always work that way.

Through the years of therapy, I was told the harder you work the farther you'll go, so I always put all of my efforts into everything I did. One of the biggest obstacles I have yet to overcome has been a reluctance to really let go of my frustrations, my fears, my anger, my sorrows, even at times my loves and joys. During the many years of therapy there were so many frustrating moments, times when I could not get my body to do what I wanted to do. There were many moments where I wanted to scream at my inabilities ... but I was always told that was not how "normal" people handled the situation.

Looking back I could see why I was told this. First, if I kept everything inside, no one but me would hurt or be hurt. When someone would/does mock me it really upset(s) me. I never did understand how people could imitate my attempts to do things, yet I knew that I always be different and not able to everything that I wanted to do.

Second, no one would have to help me deal with the problems that I would encounter. I faced a lot of ridicule from both peer and adults, and at times, I just could not handle it which later in my life led to attempted suicides. As I grew older, the ridicule became part of my life.

Last, if I kept everything inside no one would have to worry about me. My friends would not have to go through all of the emotional and mental ups and downs that would accompany me through life. Also, no one would have to experience the turmoil and confusion that my mind would/does go through.

But by keeping all these lessons in mind I am sometimes able to resist the message in Melissa

Manchester's song, DON'T CRY OUT LOUD; in which she tells people not to let go of their feelings. "DON'T CRY OUT LOUD, KEEP IT INSIDE, LEARN HOW TO HIDE YOUR FEELINGS." This is not very hard to do once you learn how to do it; but I am told by friends and professionals that work with me, I don't have to hide my emotions and that it is okay to express them, deal with them and learn to live with them. Based on my previous experiences and lessons, I now feel that expressing you feelings and emotions is a must in order to get along and survive in life.

In talking with professional people, I find that many of them feel good in learning about the frustrations and struggles that a handicapped person must go through to learn how to use his/her hands, walk, talk, and to hear; because it gives them insight to what a handicapped person must go through in order to survive. But however, there are still a few people that get their thrills by mocking and hurting someone that is a little slower in life. Not only the young must go through this, but people of all ages must endure the cruelties of society.

Now many years later since those therapy sessions have been over for me, there have been many scientific breakthroughs for the different types of handicaps; brain pacemakers, these are implanted in the brain to decrease spastic movements but would not be suitable for me because of my age, and in a few cases, cures. But it is my opinion that these "cures" often lead to false hopes. While it is true that there is a cure (relief) for some, I feel that there can never be a cure for all handicaps.

I was lucky because I did not end up in an institution like so many of the handicapped do. The following paragraphs will give you my insights and thoughts about institutions.

Many of the handicapped used to end up in an institution needlessly. When I say institution, I am emphasizing a type of facility where one must live both day and night. Also, the patients are alone by themselves most of the time. In Iowa, examples of these institutions are the Greenwood and Woodward State Hospitals. I last visited Greenwood in the early 70's, when one of my aunts was there. The patients were confined to this hospital and it seemed that they were often denied the broad range of treatments that would help them in their struggle in living. An institution provides the mere essentials and very seldom are the patients able to obtain the daily life experiences that provides one the opportunity for reaching a desired lifetime goal. Many are being treated as if it was their fault they were born different from most; and some of these patients would always require help to some degree. Many of the patients seemed to receive unfair, even cruel treatment from staff members and had to rely on the rules and the laws and the employee's degree of humanity for their care.

For some, there was also a room with "adult babies" in it where the patients stayed that needed this type of care. These patients whom the staff considered as babies would lay with only a shirt, diaper and rubber pants on just as a real baby lays when he or she is in their crib for a long period of time. These patients are also given a doll, a rattle, or a teddy bear; a pacifier, and an extra bottle to keep them "content" until someone comes to change and feed them. Therefor, being denied the quality of life.

A ll of the unjust treatments handicapped individuals receive from society are totally unnecessary. Given a chance, handicapped people such as myself and others, can be just as productive and self sufficient as non-handicapped people. For many, the only thing holding them back is their own limitations. But for many, there are ways to adjust in order to succeed through their limitations. All society really has to do is give them a fighting chance. These handicapped individuals WILL make it, through their own determination and hard work.

Dear Lord,

Please help me find the strength and courage that is
    needed to fight each and every day. I pray to You for
    Your divine help.

Amen

CHAPTER 4: SMITH-WARREN SCHOOL

S mith-Warren was the first school that was built in Ottumwa for the physically and/or mentally handicapped. The first building for this school was a two story house. The house, the special therapy equipment, furniture and staff was all financed through the funds raised from the 1954 telethon for Cerebral Palsy.

Most of the six hours that I was here everyday was spent in therapy. So my uncle Harley, as mentioned previously, was the one who taught me scholastically. He knew I was able to learn and do the work, but there was not enough hours at school for me to be taught very much.

He made sure that I kept my studies up scholastically, he even had me writing cursive writing before it was time for me to do so.

On the first floor of this house one would find the following rooms: three therapy rooms, a classroom, two bathrooms, a kitchen with a large fold down table for the students to eat at and a screened in porch. Also on first floor one would find such articles as wheelchairs, walkers, braces, crutches, canes, desks, exercise equipment and the much dreaded "relaxation" chair.

The second floor was used for staff offices.

The driveway to this school was a very steep hill and in the winter when it was icy and the City Cab, which is how the students got back and forth to school, could not make it up the driveway, the students either had to walk up the driveway and/or be carried up it. I remember that it was very hard for me to get up the hill because of my braces, but with help and determination, I usually made it. The school moved out by the Pickwick School in 1961.

I remember some of the special times, besides the telethons, that I attended or participated in while attending this school. I remember being involved with cake walks that were held twice a year to help raise money for food and supplies for the school. Also, I remember going on floats to the Halloween parties that were held at the Coliseum; I went to some of the Safety Patrol award dinners when I was a Safety Patrol person in this school; and I remember going with the other students on tours of the police station, fire station and some of the banks.

The American Legion would sponsor many of our parties and picnics, also, they would take the students to see the Circus and/or the county fair. I remember one year they took me to the Shriner Hospital in Chicago to see if they could offer more help for me; but like the doctors in Iowa City, the doctors could not offer any more help. However, they were able to help the other student that went that day.

I remember the teacher, Mrs. Hale, who was in charge of teaching fifteen students ranging from the ages of four to eighteen in one classroom. Because I was in the relaxation chair for a big portion of the day, she would tape my papers to the lap board so that I could do my work. I had the opportunity to talk to her about her memories of having me as a student in later years, which was very vague for her because she was suffering from Alzheimer's Disease, This is what she shared with me.

"I remember feeling sorry for Debbie when she first started coming to school. She would cry when her parents would leave her with strangers or the therapists would try new treatments on her.

I especially felt hurt for her when they placed her in the relaxation chair everyday; needless to say, Debbie hated that chair. Also, it took me a long time to figure out why Debbie would cry when we played music during rest time; for a long time I did not realize that the record player was too loud and hurt her ears. Debbie had hearing problems and loud noises bothered her ears." (I had trouble figuring this out also because I love music, especially country western.)

"Debbie was eager to learn and it was hard for me to keep up with her scholastic quest because

I was very limited on what I could teach her. I was very happy for her when we moved our school out next to a regular school so that Debbie had a chance to learn more. "

When I had trouble trying to do the work Mrs. Hale or Harley would help me with it. The only problems they couldn't help me with were the workbooks and writing small and neat enough to please my third and fourth grade teachers. I would get discouraged a lot but they were both there when the regular school system got to me.

Everyone whom I met while attending this school will always remain dear to me in my heart. Many of the students have passed away, some I was either by their side or holding them. I will always be a big part of this school as long as I live. May all that I knew from this school rest in eternal peace.

Unfortunately, this school was closed in the early 80's because there were not enough students left to attend here and keep the school open. I feel sad over this because I do not feel that the regular school system is for all handicapped students.

SMITH - WARREN SCHOOL

Smiling faces of the students.
Moral support for all who are there.
Ideas for the future.
Teaching is the key.
Hoping for a future.

Waiting for progress to be made.
Areas for exploring.
Ready to learn.
Relaxing is not as easy as it seems.
Exercise equipment waiting to be used.
Needing help for all your life.

Success may never come to those attending here.
Choices are very few.
Handicaps are definitely present.
Omitting defeat is not always possible.
Only a few dreams can come true.
Lord, we all really need Your grace to survive.

Deb

CHAPTER 5: MAIN STREAMING ME INTO PICKWICK SCHOOL

The fall of 1963, my second year of third grade, I was purposely held back so that I could be mainstreamed and with kids close to my age, is when I would begin the main streaming experiment. I was entering a system that was not totally accessible architecturally wise and the work may prove to be too much for me, but I was willing to give it a try. I was to be the first severely handicapped student to be mainstreamed and the road ahead of me would not be an easy one; yet if I succeeded, other handicapped students would be able to attend the regular school system. It was rough, but I succeeded with my efforts and determination.

I would attend Pickwick for a half day during third and fourth grade and all day during fifth and sixth grade. In third and fourth grade I would still get three hours of therapy in the afternoon; and during fifth and sixth grade, I would have therapy during gym class.

My teacher, therapists, and the school board felt that it was time for me to have the chance to learn as much as possible. I had gone through all of the learning materials that Smith-Warren had. I would not have an easy time with my new surroundings because I had never been in a classroom where I was the only handicapped student before, and I was VERY scared.

Not only would I feel peer pressure and ridicule, but I would endure the fact that some of my teachers would be very uneasy having me in class. For many of the teachers, I was the only handicapped student that they had at this point of time. Let's begin my experiment now.

Upon walking into the classroom on the first day of the school year, I felt very frightened and nervous of my surroundings. I was so scared that after I was introduced to Mrs. Ryan, I took a seat in the back of the room. There was a lot of ridicule and pressure during this year, but I could not discuss it with the students at Smith-Warren because they could not understand why I was attending a different school. My therapists and Mrs. Hale became concerned when they saw the pressure getting to me but they wanted me to have the chance to learn as much as possible. I knew I could talk about my problems and frustrations, but they also knew I had to stick it out.

I remember the third day of school that year when Mrs. Ryan called me to the front of the room, in front of everyone, when it was time for penmanship class. I could not write small and neat yet, so staying in the small lines of the paper was not easy for me to do. Mrs. Ryan announced in front of the entire class that she wanted me to take my writing lessons on the blackboard since I could not write small and neatly on paper. However, after seeing how hard it was to erase my work, Mrs. Ryan scolded me about writing too hard for the board to be easily erased. I could not win that day no matter how hard I tried. I was glad when noon came so I could return to Smith-Warren. It really hurt when she and the class laughed at me that day.

Upon my return to Smith-Warren, I did not go into the lunchroom to eat but went to my classroom instead. Miss Hendrix waited for awhile to see if I was coming to lunch, when I didn't she came down to the classroom to see why. I explained to her how my morning had gone. The two of us talked about it and she finally persuaded me to eat. The next day before I arrived Miss Hendrix walked over to talk to Mrs. Ryan about the events of the previous day, this only made matters worse. I was startled at the increased ridicule that day, but I kept plugging away at it for the rest of the year.

Mr. Black, the principal, checked two weeks later and noticed that I was still being made to take my writing lessons on the blackboard; the teacher was fired at the end of the school year. I was glad when that year of nightmares was over!

Fourth grade with Mrs. Carr would be similar at first, but as the year progressed she began to accept me and my efforts of doing the work. Mrs. Carr had seen me the year before so she knew the challenges that she was up against. I remember one trying winter day when Mrs. Carr seemed to be at her worst. Upon my arrival, I gave her my workbook as I had done every day since the start of the year. When she opened the book and saw that the writing wasn't any smaller, she blew up. This is the conversation that took place.

"Debbie, I really do not see how you expect me to read this. Why can't you write as small as the other students? Better yet, why do even try when you know that you can't do the work? I honestly do not know what the School Board was thinking when they had you come to this school."

I was startled at her remarks because she had not blown up at me before. I told her that I was doing my best.

"Well try harder" was her reply.

Even though it was snowing and cold when recess came that day, I went out to get some fresh air and to have time to think; this was not the case though as Mrs. Carr was the teacher in charge of recess that day. She came over and started screaming at me for coming out in the cold, then she resumed her lecture about my writing. When I went back inside, I tried to please her for the rest of the morning.

I had to miss a week of going over to Pickwick in fourth grade because I had fallen and sprained my ankle. I was using a wheelchair at Smith-Warren because I couldn't walk and I knew that I would not be able to get around at Pickwick in a wheelchair. I was taken off guard when I found out that she did not know what happened because I had been given my assignments. In fact she was surprised and pleased when she opened my workbooks and saw how neat they were. She asked me who did the writing for me;

I told her I did but under less pressure. Needless to say, Mrs. Carr was happy to get my work for the rest of the year.

At the end of the year Mrs. Carr took the class on a picnic at Wildwood Park and she asked me to join the class in going. Because I was also going to Smith - Warren part of the day, I had to get permission from the school board and Smith - Warren as well as my parents; but I did get to go and felt as if I belonged there. The games that the class played were similar to the ones I had seen them play during recess. I joined in where possible and I was happy that day. By working very hard that year, I made a lot of progress that Mrs. Carr did not feel I would ever make. At the picnic she told me how happy and proud she was of me. She also told me that she hoped I would achieve my attempts in doing whatever I tried to do. I finished fourth grade with a happy feeling in my heart.

Fifth grade was a new experience for me. The school at this level was departmentalized so that the students could get used to having more than one teacher for everything. I would start learning how to move from class to class with a congestion of students. It was here that full main streaming began for me; I only went to Smith - Warren for therapy while the rest of the class took physical education. At first the class had trouble understanding why I wasn't in gym class with them, but after seeing me make a little more progress, they accepted the fact.

I can remember the first day of school that year when the principal and my physical therapist walked into the classroom with me, we kind of took the teacher by surprise. Mrs. Black had taken roll call and she thought that all of her students were present. When Mr. Smith, the principal, called her name she looked up with an expression of shock on her face. Mr. Smith introduced me and explained that I would be in her class then he and Mr. Jarvis left.

After getting seated, Mrs. Black asked if I would be attending classes there all day or half a day. I remember that she seemed genuinely pleased that she would be working with me full time. Also during the first week of being a full time student, Mr. Smith arranged for me to ride the country bus home so that my parents would not have to pick me up and it gave me some time for myself along with the opportunity for some of the students to accept me. The bus went by the store every day so it was arranged for me to get off there.

Spring is a busy time for those in school. Everyone is trying to get all of their work caught up so they can pass to the next grade; as well as singing in school concerts, making projects for the art show, outings and so forth. Upon returning from therapy one afternoon I was told about the art show where students had the opportunity displaying their work. I had came back from therapy with a woven rug that I had made. Mrs. Black fell in love with it and asked me to enter it in the art show since I had been unable to make any of the art projects by myself. I agreed to do so. Unfortunately my family did not like the idea and I was severely punished for it. After the art show, Mrs. Black told me if it had been made in her classroom I would have won first prize; but because the rug had been made off of school grounds, she and the other judges could not judge it fairly against the other students work. Nevertheless, I was overjoyed with her praise.

I remember one day of this year when I fell and hurt my back. I was outside during recess playing with some friends, Kim, Betsy, and Jessica, at recess when I fell. Perhaps we got a little rough. Because I was able to get up by myself at the time, my friends and I did not get worried about the possibility of me being hurt. In fact, because I was not in pain or anything, I did not think I was really hurt bad. The first thought that went through my mind was that I was going to be paralyzed again. Most people were/are amazed that I remember anything about not being able to move; but I can remember because I wanted to be able to escape the abuse, and this meant I had to be able to move.

I thought I was going to have to ask Mrs. Black to call over to Smith - Warren and ask Mr. Jarvis to bring over a wheelchair in order for me to get to my next class. I was afraid of what might happen at home, so I kept trying to get up on my own until I finally made it up. My back continued hurting for a long time and I eventually had to seek medical attention for it, which made my parents very angry with me, but I was very fortunate that there was no serious injury.

In 1980, I contacted Mrs. Black to ask her to write a summary of what she remembered about having me in class. She was always a thoughtful person and didn't tell me that she was dying of Cancer at the time; she died two years later, hence the brevity of her account. Mrs. Black played an important role during fifth and sixth grade, thus I include her vague yet remarkable memories.

"Debbie, it has been so long ago that I can't remember anything. I remember your penmanship and how you worked at it. As for Social Studies, I can't remember what I taught you, but I know you were a good student."

"I remember one day when you returned to school after being very ill, I had a sore throat and you were very kind to give me one of your cough drops. It really helped. I've brought that kind every since."

Also in fifth and sixth grades, we took a Spanish class from a tv course. It was very hard for me to do, but when the teacher came to visit our class, I was able to carry a conversation with him.

I finished fifth grade pretty well scholastically, but there were many frustrating moments for me. I had to work hard in order for me to learn, but I eventually realized that I could learn like my peers.

Mrs. Norris, who was mainly a sixth grade teacher, was who I had for Science and Spelling in fifth and sixth grades. She was also my home room teacher in sixth grade.

We were very busy in sixth grade. As a Science project my class went on a tour of the public

Waterworks. Because I walked slower, Paula, my sister, went with us so that Mrs. Norris could stay with the rest of the class. There were six hundred steps to climb to reach the roof of the waterworks, Mrs. Norris understood when I did not join them there.

Also, we made a trip to Evans Junior High School, which is where I would go if I was lucky, Mr. Jarvis went with me so he could see how the school was set up and help me through the lunch line. I learned that I would have steps to go up and down and I would have to pace myself a little faster. Also, I learned that the teachers were a little bit more prepared for me, but there would be a lot more ridicule.

Another experience that I remember is the day Mrs. Norris entered my math class and asked me to take a walk with her. At first, I was a little scared and confused, then she told me the school nurse wanted to talk to me. When I first entered her office, I kept asking myself what I did wrong. The nurse needed some information regarding what special considerations were needed at school and about my general health to send over to the school nurse. During the forty-five minutes that we talked, she explained to me that the main streaming experiment was going to get harder. I thought at the time I could handle the pressure, but as you will see later, I did not always do a very good job at it.

The following lines are from Mrs. Norris.

"As I reflect upon the many boys and girls that have been welcomed in my class, one special girl comes to mind. Although physically handicapped, she willingly met each new challenge with a smile and an apparent desire to win."

"She never permitted her limited abilities to interfere with her classroom activities. This young lady graciously accepted the reality of her physical abilities."

"Her persistent effort for achievement was well accepted by her fellow classmates, who in turn, endeavored to assist her in any manner they could."

"It was a rewarding experience to be associated with and teach Debbie. It is my feeling that our lives have been enriched by this experience."

The next person to share their thoughts with me was Mrs. Allen, another teacher that I had in fifth and sixth grade.

"When I had Debbie in my class, I sincerely believe that I gained as much or perhaps even more than she did from this experience. We were split up into departments at this school and my area was Language Arts. She was also in the group I had for Reading each day. Every child is a distinct person and personality, but naturally I was especially concerned about Debbie and was fully aware of the ultimate effort it must have been for her in trying to adjust and succeed in such demanding circumstances. Just getting materials gathered and moving from class to class was difficult at times."

"In Language class, there was a great deal of work that required writing. She always fulfilled each assignment, not asking for, or expecting any favors. I appreciated her understanding and patience with those who worked with her. It seems to me she had marvelous insight with her peers and with adults. Her work was always commendable and totally acceptable grade - wise."

In 1987, two fellow classmates, Shelly Howell and Amy Hill, shared a few of their thoughts with me. The first is from Shelly.

"I first met Debbie in third or fourth grade at the Pickwick Elementary School. She was very pretty with dark brown hair and even darker brown eyes, the type that reflect the light and sun to glisten. She was physically impaired in the following ways: her speech was slurred, she could not control her saliva, she shook all over constantly, she had great difficulty walking, and she was a great deal taller than the other kids her age."

"Debbie was very kind and friendly, but often kids would not try to get to know her; I suppose now that they feared the unknown. She also had occasional problems with teachers who did not want to take the time to understand what she was saying or could not read what she had written."

"I hurt so much for Debbie at the time. Why would God do this to such a wonderful and innocent human being? I remember Debbie crying because she would try so hard and get so frustrated. No matter what, Debbie never gave up."

"I remember going to Debbie's thirteenth birthday party. I got her an autograph animal so all her friends could sign it. She was so happy that day."

"We are all grown up now and in the same Literature class in college. Debbie no longer has a lot of trouble controlling her saliva, talks clearer, and we are about the same height now. I'm glad Debbie never gave up trying or she could never have come this far."

"I didn't know until recently that Debbie is also impaired mentally. Shr told me that the back half of her brain is dead. That being so, look how much she achieved. She has learned with half as much what we have trouble learning with all. I am so proud of her."

"After all the obstacles Debbie has conquered, she seems very depressed instead of proud. I don't know what is troubling her. Whatever it is, it seems that it is her turn to be happy, so God, please help Debbie work through her problems. You owe her a good turn."

The following is what Amy had to share.

"Debbie told me that she was mainstreamed at the Pickwick Elementary School when she was in third grade. I first attended Pickwick in fourth grade Debbie and I were in the same home room in sixth grade."

"I recall two specific situations involving Debbie. In a sixth grade class our teacher selected team captains to choose teammates for an educational game. I was a captain and remember choosing Debbie early in the selection process because I knew she was intelligent and her handicap did not affect her intellectual capacity."

"Another recollection is being invited to Debbie's thirteenth birthday party. My friends and I were apprehensive about the situation since we had never been with Debbie outside of the school setting or met her family. We were all a little nervous about attending her party, but realized how important the party would be to Debbie and we wanted to treat her as any other classmate."

"I don't really remember what kind of introduction students received when Debbie was in class. I feel an explanation of her handicap, its cause and limitations, would have been helpful to students. I'm sure classmates would have presumed she was mentally retarded, but those sharing classes with her were soon aware that she was not handicapped mentally."

From those grade school days so many of my teachers and classmates walk with me still, and faces for the most part are lost to me today. Yet their kindness lives on in me whenever a stranger holds the door open a second longer, or offers to carry a burden of books for me in college, or just be friendly toward me now that I'm out of school. Their cruelties remain also, perhaps refined and less obvious, but still there in a stare, a jibe, or even in the faces of those who don't seem to se or hear me. I once had to fight social ridicule by demonstrating that I could do what everyone else did, but in a different way. Today, I can ignore the ridicule and keep moving forward.

CHAPTER 6: EVANS JUNIOR HIGH SCHOOL

This school is where I began to really feel the pressure of making the experiment work. Along with the abuse was the pressure of certain required classes and class work and the increase of peer ridicule. It was hard enough to keep up with my studies, but some of my classes were at an advanced level. Remember if you can, I was at a higher intellectual level than I was movement wise. I did the work but I always felt like a failure.

I compensated my failures by attempting suicide for the first time at the age of thirteen. I did this by taking overdoses of aspirin and other over the counter medications. I would use some of my prescription medicines later in life. The only thing I accomplished at the time was to ruin my health. I would keep trying to kill myself for a LONG time because I wanted to die to escape the pains of school and abuse.

The peer pressure increased more at this school; so much that three boys, who would later be my friends, were caught tripping me on the steps. I just felt that I was falling more because the crowd was bigger and I had to hurry more to get to my classes. When the boys were caught the principal made them apologize to me before expelling them for the entire year from school. Naturally, his actions did not set well with the other students and I was blamed for their being expelled. Upon their return to school, they had an entire different attitude towards me.

Also, this is where I first tried taking Gym which was required for each student to take at the time. Mrs. Running, the Gym teacher, came down to my home room to talk to me about taking the course after I had let the office know that I could not participate in this class. Mrs. Running told me that she felt that the activities could be adapted enough for me to participate in the class. I proved that I could not handle this class. Between Gym, class work, and peer ridicule, I developed some serious health problems, and this made taking the course more impossible for me. Although it hurt when the other students would laugh at my attempts in Gym, I had the satisfaction knowing that I gave it my best shot.

Eighth grade had two events that stand out in my mind. First, every girl is required to take Homemaking in eighth grade. Of course there as the BIG question of rather I would be able to do the requirements ofthe course. Toward the end of the curse the teachersthat tauht ticourse did a series of tests on me that involved the activities of the class. Through these tests the teachers reached the decision that I should sign up for the class. When I went to start this class, I found that I was assigned to the Vice Principal's office, which the other students though I had gotten in trouble was why I was there, by a decision that the School Administration made over the summer. The Administration felt the class had too many safety risks for me, so I was given the extra time for studying. After I left Pickwick, the School Board was always trying to put me in the special education classes, but the teachers did not feel that this was where I belonged.

The other special event was being nominated Teen of the month. Each home room would nominate someone to represent each grade and one month my class had nominated me. I was sick when they took the vote so the teacher read the write - up about me to the class upon my return. I was really a part of them now! I did not win the nomination but I was happy to hear that my peers were starting to accept me.

Ninth grade was to offer a challenge that I was very uncomfortable with. In Geography class each student was to select a chapter and teach that chapter to the class. For most students this was an honor, but for me it would possibly be another nightmare experience; fortunately the students proved me wrong and it was a learning experience for the entire class. Needless to say, I did NOT want to do this and asked if I could do something else instead. Of course, I was told no. I was nervous but my work for my chapter was done. Along with discussing the chapter, each student along with the supervision of the teacher, was responsible for making study sheets and a test for the class. When I was due to teach, the teacher was out ill and I was on my own. I made a few mistakes, but I thought I handled the situation well.

Also in ninth grade it was necessary for me to be evaluated in Iowa City at the Hospital School to see if it would be humanly possible for me to attend high school in Ottumwa. Scholastically there was no question but physically, the high school had over five hundred steps to be climbed daily; there were other architectural barriers also which raised another safety issue. After taking therapy treatments in Iowa City for the summer, the doctors agreed to let me return home for school with the understand that I would return in six months for an evaluation AND spend the next summer at the Hospital School. Needless to say but my parents did not follow through with the agreement.

While at Evans I met Rebecca Hayes, Ellen Myers and Brian Burke. Rebecca and Ellen are both Registered Nurses and School Nurses. For a long time Rebecca and I were close friends until later years when problems arose between us. Brian is a School Social Worker who I met during a time of personal troubles. We used to keep pretty close tabs on each other, but in 1974 when I told him that my Vocational Rehabilitation files were being closed because my parents could not agree on any of the programs being offered to me, we drifted apart for awhile. And we probably should have stayed apart because he seemed more on my parents side than mine. Brian helped me to learn how to make friends and tried to get me to stay out of psychological trouble; we did not know at this time that I suffered from Organic Chemical Depression and Borderline Personality Disorders due to my CP. However it took a long time for Brian to convince me. The following paragraphs are from Brian.

"I find this task difficult to begin. On the one hand, it seems as though I have known Debbie but such a brief time ... an hour here, a telephone call there ... time always seeming too short and incomplete. On the other hand, it seems as I have always known Debbie. That's the way Debbie is."

"In fact, I first met Debbie when she was attending Evans Junior High School. In my role as a School Social Worker, it was believed that I might be of some assistance to her because of problems which ultimately needed to be shared with her family. At first glance the matter seemed rather routine, but then, nothing is very routine about Debbie. Together we decided that perhaps we could meet on a weekly basis ... one hour ... so that we could discuss her problems and encourage her to share her problems with her parents [I don't think Brian believed me about the abuse] and provide her with a measurement of support for her accomplishments."

"As a result of our time together, I enjoyed the unique opportunity to see a part of the world through Debbie's eyes. As she progressed in school ... high school and college ... our relationship intensified, no longer consumed with working on day to day problems of living and not trying to kill herself, but rather focusing on Debbie's many strengths. This was a rewarding period for me because I witnessed her coming of age, demonstrating much courage and newly found skills in her abilities to relate well with people her own age."

"Always since I first knew her, Debbie had considerable skills in being able to relate to adults. But to see her bravely conquer her fears and handle the ridicule from some of her peers was gratifying and personally rewarding ... and I believe to Debbie as well. Together Debbie and I developed a plan which would enable her to develop new friendships and maintain old ones. Basically the plan called for a series of steps to be accomplished on a weekly basis, one step at a time. Debbie's job was to keep a diary of her attempts to develop more social skills. First, the plan called for Debbie to initiate smiles and give a more pleasant appearance. "

"Second, she was to initiate greetings such as "Hi" whenever appropriate. These were not as easy to accomplish as it seems. Within the setting of busy and crowded hallways, frequently Debbie had all she could do to keep from getting knocked down without attempting eye contact and smile at whomever would give her a glance. No matter what, she would always have problems walking. However, Debbie tried very hard and succeeded enough to have gained enough confidence in her own abilities." This was one accomplishment I felt would never take place, I had many doubts for a long time in regards to the other students accepting me.

"Next, we planned for her to learn some of her classmates' names. To accomplish this would require Debbie to pay close attention to the social interactions all about her. Again she succeeded. Then the task became one of encouraging her to use the names she had learned whenever she could. Throughout this process, Debbie made remarkable progress in acquiring new friends."

"Finally, we concentrated on leaning on her ability to make "small talk" and together we would practice things she could talk to her peers about ... Friday night football games to the possibilities of going to college. Throughout this whole experience, Debbie kept track of her progress and was encouraged by her gains. Although some problems continued to exist, perhaps the biggest change I noticed was the change in Debbie's attitude about herself. No longer did she avoid people expecting to be rejected. But she became energetic about making things happen for herself. Granted, not every social contact with her peers was successful, occasionally, there was much pain."

"The super part of what Debbie did, in my estimation, she kept plugging away at it. She tried, tried, and tried again. She had to deal with people who felt sorry for her ... people who were afraid of her ... people who were uncomfortable with her ... and each new experience was a learning experience for her and for them. As a result of her attitude change, there were definite changes within her group which suggests that she caused the attitude of others to be changed about her."

"When I think about Debbie, a host of other people come to mind. Throughout her high school years and beyond, Rebecca Hayes was a very special person in Debbie's life. Without question, Debbie showed excellent judgement in choosing her for a friend and confident. Whenever Debbie needed a friend, it seemed that Rebecca was there. Such friends are rare. But in my opinion, anyone having a friend like

Rebecca is rich beyond belief ... and Debbie's rich - - rich."

"Another person whom frequently comes to mind is Debbie's father, Peter. Peter knows everybody! And he likes everybody. When I first met Peter, he was busy for a local telethon for Cerebral Palsy. Now that was at a time when the telethon was a major production ... and not the way it is now. Believe me, Peter was always in the middle of things, not only on Debbie's behalf, but anyone who was afflicted with the disease. [Father did fight for the handicapped but he came across as being a "big shot" to everyone!] He was also the kind of man who didn't take novocaine when he had a tooth pulled."

"Debbie's mom, Megan, seemed to take life for what it is. [Boy, was Brian WRONG!] She and Peter have gone through some pretty rough times, but together they have came through these rough times and survived. Debbie's sister, Paula used to be very close to her, but that seemed to change when Paula got married in 1977."

Brian was right, most of my fellow classmates did learn to accept me. But there have been many experiences with society that made me wonder at times if all my efforts were worth it. Even today I still have mixed feelings when I go out in public, but through my friends, I fight the struggle and have the courage to withstand the harassment I must deal with from other people.

CHAPTER 7: OTTUMWA HIGH SCHOOL

This was the final public school which was involved in the main streaming experiment. I did not know if I could pass the test here because there were over five hundred steps to climb several times a day. Even after practicing a lot at the Hospital School could not prepare me for my daily battle. I was able to walk but my body was starting the process of going downhill without my knowing it. Steps was/is a serious problem for me because of my tendency to fall easily.

The next three years would be a rough and hard time but with much encouragement from many people, I was able to come out ahead of my problems. Along with fighting the stairs, there were many academic activities that I needed help with. In Biology for an example, I needed help in preparing the slides and doing the experiments. In some of the other classes it was necessary for the teachers to enlarge the lines of the workbooks for me. I was able to write more neatly, but it was still difficult for me to write on fine - lined paper.

Everyone tried to help me when the going got rough, but sometimes I was the only one who could work things out. I met a lot of students and teachers here, but I also had the philosophy that my studies came first before anything else. Maybe if I had given some time to recreation, I never went out while I was attending school, I might not have had so much trouble making friends. By this time I was so used to the abuse that my studies didn't suffer so much. I was able to make the honor roll several times.

Some special memories of high school years really stick out in my mind. First, the local Cerebral Palsy Association purchased an electric typewriter so that it would be easier for me to do my assignments. I did not realize at the time that the typewriter would be mine to keep. That's how dumb I was.

I have always had trouble writing because of my hands shaking all the time, so the typewriter eliminated many frustrating moments and made everything I did easier to read. Another problem I had/have with writing is that I needed to hold my hand and lean on my arm for stability to make the work clear. Many people was embarrassed by this, some even thought I was playing with my breast; no that was NOT the case.

Second, I would follow the floats downtown. The floats were made as a part of the Homecoming activities. I never had an interest in football, but I enjoyed looking at the floats.

As a part of my study halls in my junior year, it was arranged for me to work in the Audio Visual Department. Along with my cleaning responsibilities, I had the chance to learn what was all done in this department. Also, in my senior year, I assisted the Sociology teachers in recording grades in the grade book. Although I did not get credit for doing these things, it was a learning experience for me.

During my senior year, I had to make some trips to Iowa City for some dental work to be done.

Because of the fact there was so much work to be done, my dentist felt it would be best for the work to be done to me in the hospital. The actual work, which was started by pulling three of my teeth, began one and a half weeks before the Christmas vacation started. I had many problems with bleeding from my gums, and at this time we found out I was a bleeder.

What was only to be a two day absence, ended up to be a total of three weeks. I bled for two and a half of the three weeks! This time included our regular vacation. I was still pretty pale when I went back to school; the teachers and Rebecca was pretty worried. Rebecca had seen me over Christmas to exchange gifts, but she didn't expect for me to still be so pale. It didn't help that Rebecca came back with a bad cold and she was scared that I would catch it. I was still very weak from losing so much blood, so Rebecca and my Uncle Harley worried even more until they started to see signs of my health coming back. Harley told Rebecca he had been worried ever since he saw me at Christmas, and that didn't help matters.

The rest of the work, which was a lot of filling and capping my teeth, was completed one week after graduation. My graduation money, which was really meant to be spent on me, was used to pay for my sister, mother and grandmother on mother's side, to stay in a hotel, the Colonial Inn, which was one of the most expensive hotels. I would not have minded so much if I had been asked instead of told about the situation! Needless to say, there was no money left over for me to spend. I was in surgery for seven and a half hours; it was only supposed to be a three to three and a half surgery. Once I was in surgery, the doctors had trouble saving my teeth by just filling them, so they had to cap several of them.

My saliva seemed to rot my teeth no matter what I did. Instead of wasting the money to have my teeth filled all of the time, I had my teeth pulled and started wearing upper dentures in July 1989. I have had a new set of dentures since, but as was always predicted, it is very hard for me to keep the lower ones in, and this makes a few people very frustrated with me.

While I was in high school, I had the chance to work with Vocational Rehabilitation. The different programs that were being offered to me didn't work out because my parents refused to give their permission for me to participate in them. For instance, my counselor wanted to send me to Camp Sunnyside's Homebound Training Program. This program trains the individual different craft skills, then once at home, they help the individual to obtain the needed equipment to work with so they can earn some money. Another program that my parents did not agree with was the evaluation at Oakdale; it was decided through this evaluation, that I would be best suited in a sheltered workshop.

The most important event however was Graduation. I don't know who was the proudest – my family and friends or me. But I do know that I will cherish that night forever. I was very proud and happy to think that I was able to graduate with the rest of my class. I was given a seat in the front row so that I would not have to walk so far. The only part of graduation that I did not get to participate in was the walk around the field; instead Harley walked me across the field to my seat. But he forgot to come for me after the activities so I was on my own to get back to the top. There was a party for the seniors after graduation was over, but I didn't go due to family obligations.

May my memories and mistakes of school years remain with me forever. Yet, let me learn from them and proceed in bettering my life the best way possible. The following thoughts are from Mrs. Darling, "Chief," one of my high school teachers.

"When Debbie, as a sophomore, first came into my class, she was withdrawn and insecure; after I learned that I was being transferred to this class, some, especially my parents and sister, told me that it was a class for dummies, rather that associate with her peers would seek my attention. Most of her previous friends were adults and/or other handicapped people. No wonder, then, that our massive and less - than - understanding student body seemed so alien and hostile to her. "

"At first, I went along with Debbie's dependency on me. Then it began to dawn on me that Debbie had to get on her own two feet and begin fighting for some of the dreams and goals she wanted from life. My patronizing attitude was not helping her to believe in her own powers."

"I had to be firm; and at times, I may have seemed cruel, but Debbie began to develop a more positive attitude." All during my life I have had to prove to people that I was not retarded, in many cases, I was not successful in doing so.

"During the next two years, Debbie showed more and more progress, more optimism. This does not mean that Debbie had or has attained her goals. But she was and is on her way. It has been a long trip, it will always be a long trip, so much further than you and I will ever have to go." Mrs. Darling talks about the long trip that I have had in life, and I can't help wondering if everyone that faces a trip because of a handicap feels at times the journey is not worth it.

CHAPTER 8: OTTUMWA HEIGHTS COLLEGE

After high school I went to college at Ottumwa Heights in Ottumwa for a year. I wanted to pursue my life long dream of becoming a Librarian. Scholastically I was not qualified to be a student but spiritually this was something I really wanted. I was accepted as a student, but I was placed on probation. Vocational Rehabilitation and the Cerebral Palsy Association provided all of the funding for me to attend classes here. The pressure of getting high grades was just too much for me.

The college was ran by the Sisters of Humanity and they had very specific guidelines for the students. I was not Catholic and I wasn't as smart as most of the students, but the Sisters were willing to give me a chance. When my advisor became ill in the middle of the Fall semester, the Sisters tried everything to help me so I could stay in school. However, it just wasn't meant to be. I was trying to help several family members as well as going to school; I learned that I couldn't do several things at once.

Along with classes it was required for students to attend the parties. To please everyone, I went to the Halloween party as a farmer. I did not enjoy it though knowing that I needed to be studying every minute that I could. At Christmastime the Sisters had a candle light banquet for all of the students. I was not going to go but some of the staff really wanted me to go. Paula was working in the infirmary, so the Sisters enlisted her help in persuading me to go. When the Sisters figured out the real reason I did not want to go, everything was taken care of for me. They even arranged the date with a boy, Sean, for me. Reluctantly, I gave in and went.

Sean told me during dinner that he would not be returning for the Spring semester because his grades were not good enough. I was confused about this because my grades wasn't any better. When I asked about this, I was told that my grades had came up a little and the teachers wanted to give me a chance, but Sean had not shown any improvement. I felt sorry for Sean but didn't know how to help him.

I kept trying to get better grades the following semester, but it just wasn't meant to be. In my heart I had failed and there was nothing anyone could do for me. I dropped out of school at the end of the semester and tried to care for and help my family as much as possible.

CHAPTER 9: THE IN BETWEEN EVENTS AND THOUGHTS OF THE FIRSTTWENTY YEARS OF MY LIFE

I want to now share some things that helped shape me while I was growing up. Please remember that I had to deal with a disability, depression, and abuse of some sort from day one. A part of abuse was neglect because my parents did not want to admit that I belong to them. However, there was good times too.

Most people thought we were a close knit family, but in reality we were never that close. Because of my depression, I allowed myself to please people by doing whatever they wanted done and not allowing myself to do what I wanted to do.1959 was to begin the years of hardship for my family, but we went through each day the best we could. Peter, my father, was working at the John Morrell packing plant when he hurt his back and would never be able to do hard labor again. He fell on a piece of fat that had fallen on the floor with seven hundred pounds of fat in his arms. He damaged several vertebras which would require two back surgeries; but the damage was permanent and work was out of the question, so the financial worries began.

Naturally father did not believe in living off Welfare programs and he became very angry when he had to resort to them. So when he could move around a little, he worked at odd jobs such as electrical and plumbing. Also he would repair fans and lawnmowers for people. Later he took over the grocery store so that my grandparents could retire; but grandma would help out whenever she could.

Summer of 1959 was especially rough for mother. Father was in Chicago attending a rehabilitation center, I was in Iowa City getting use to new leg braces and having a broken arm taken care of which I got after a fall, and Paula was at home recuperating from a broken leg which she received after falling off of her bicycle. Father was in hopes of getting the proper training so that he could go back to work, unfortunately that was not the case.

The holiday season of 1959 was special for my family. We had decided to forget about Christmas, but the employees of the packing plant had other plans for us; they knew we had no money coming in except for what they collected each month to help us with bills. Christmas Eve there was a knock on the door, we opened the door to find a line of cars and trucks on the street. Each car and truck was filled with food and presents for the family. Everyone knew we couldn't give anything in return, yet they knew their help was appreciated.

In 1962, I attended Camp Sunnyside for the first time. The camp was sponsored by Easter Seals and private donations. One would find every type of handicap here but it was a place where the campers did not have to worry about what other people thought. I would attend through a camper scholarship and I had a lot of fun.

I remember 1963 when I got to take my braces off for good. I did not complain about wearing them but there were days when they seemed to weigh three times their actual weight; I really don't know how much they did weigh because everyone kept giving me different numbers for their weight. I did not mind wearing them because I knew eventually they would help me.

I remember that in the late 60's we went to Kansas for a wedding. It was hot but we camped out in the car at night because there wasn't any extra money for hotel rooms. We ended up seeing the entire state in the time we were there. Our relatives had a hard time accepting this and wanted to give us extra money to get home on, but father said no because he didn't want to owe anybody and keep what pride and dignity he had left. Needless to say, the relatives would not take no for an answer and it caused problems with the relatives and my father.

I remember that several of the relatives lived along the way on our way home and they all insisted that we stop. At each stop we were greeted with a meal, Paula and I had trouble eating so much that we had to say no a lot. Someone would borrow the car and took it to fill it up with gas, oil, food, and drinks. Each time father got mad, but everyone seemed to use the excuse and reminder that there were two minors in the car and they wanted to help us all. By the time we got home we had a week's supply of groceries; and the next day there was a delivery from Kansas with enough food, cleaning supplies, and money to last us six months. I never saw father get so mad at people on the phone as I did that day. Again my father told everyone off for trying to help.

I was baptized on February 14, 1965. Although I was not quite the age our church baptizes its members, our minister allowed me to baptized the same day my mother and sister were. He knew that I was ready to accept Christ into my life. Being baptized signified that I was ready to accept and obey the ways of Jesus. It also shows that one is ready to worship the Lord through fellowship with others. Through this fellowship, I was able to express my love, faith and respect for others. In 1965, my parents took over ownership of the Hang Out. I'll talk about it more later.

In 1970, I returned to camp. I made my knitting board by hand and I have gotten a lot of use out of it.

CHAPTER 10: LIFE GOES ON

My parents had owned and operated The Hang Out from 1965 - 1984, but it had been in the family since 1949. At one time the store had been a one room tavern and we expanded it through the years to the equivalent to four rooms. I remember when Paula and I were younger, we helped out in the store. In the early days there had been auction sales and/or dances in the garage out back, and this is where I really got to help. When Paula cashiered the sales, I got to carry the sheets to her. We continued to work more and more as Paula and I grew older. After the store closed in 1984, I used the building and/or garage for rummage sales, craft sales, and a place to use my electric typewriter so that it wouldn't get on anyone's nerves. I would work there until I left home in 1987.

By working in the store, I was able to demonstrate to the public that the handicapped CAN work. For a long time society viewed the handicapped as contagious, retarded, or unable to work. I proved that theory wrong. During the 80's, the decade of the handicapped, society was able to see more and more of the handicapped out in public places such as schools, businesses, and out on the job market. On a personal basis, I was no longer asked "Are you contagious?" I could easily tell people that they would not get a handicap just by being around someone who has a handicap. I feel I no longer have to hide because I'm different.

The store provided me with a way to educate people by showing them that a handicapped person could overcome adversity with hopes of a better tomorrow. I was able to overcome my fears of the way people thought of me and I would eventually return to school.

After I left college in 1974, I practically took care of the business as my parents were starting to have health problems. Most of the customers knew me and understood that it might take a little longer to be waited on. Friends and relatives could come here and visit and/or have a meal with us and not feel out of place. I surprised and worried many friends when I no longer thought of myself or a future so I could take care of everyone. I helped my grandmother on my father's side as well as caring for my family. With both parents and grandmother ill, and my sister "needed" help caring for her son and keeping her house clean, I felt that all of the responsibility fell on my shoulders, both physically and financially.

We officially closed the store in 1984, but it was not put in the paper until August 31, 1985. The reasons for the closing was a lack of business because you could get groceries cheaper at the supermarkets than we could wholesale, and my parent's health was getting worse. While my parents were sorting what they wanted to keep from what they wanted to sell, they used the building as a gathering place and as a place to hold year round rummage sales.

After we closed the store I decided to return to college. I wanted to get the proper help to finish my book and pursue a career, which I was unable to get a job because of my handicap. I left Ottumwa in 1988 to pursue a life of my own.

SERIOUS TIMES HIT THE FAMILY

In 1977, father had a massive coronary heart attack at the age of fifty and we almost lost him.

Later that year on October 17, he had open heart surgery, it was necessary to replace the three main arteries and the main vein going to his heart. He never felt well after that. In 1986 Iowa City wanted to do another surgery, but because there was no guarantee that he would feel better, father said no. Another reason father said no is the doctors told us he wouldn't make it through the surgery. He was now totally disabled and eligible for Social Security, because I am handicapped and considered as a dependent, I was also able to receive benefits. Father died May 29, 1992.

In 1978 people were starting to worry more about me. I was no longer happy and it seemed that I had just given up. My case worker had met with me secretly, or so we thought, and tried to help me get out of my home life. Once my family found out, all hell broke loose. Needless to say, it was another nine years before I was able to leave the situation. The worker, is now the coordinator of the services that I receive; she may be two hours away, but when there is trouble, she is there for me.

In 1979, mother fell and hurt her arm after falling in the mud while chasing my nephew. She ended up having to stay in the hospital for a few days because the fall had caused her sugar count to go sky high so they taught her how to take insulin. Mother was a brittle diabetic which made healing even more difficult. No matter what she did, mother could not get her sugar under control.

On January 27, 1980, it was my turn. I did not go to the hospital but it was the beginning of my having constant pain in my legs and lower back, and there would not be a medical answer to why I have/had this pain. I woke up in the middle of the night and my left leg was doubled up under me. It took three long hours to straighten my leg out, after getting it straightened out I had trouble using it because of the pain. Within a week, the pain was in both legs and I had trouble walking from the pain, however I kept pushing myself daily until May 1988, when I started using an electric wheelchair. I knew that it was serious because the only time that I really feel my body is when I am in pain. Some days the pain was/is worse than others but a person can learn to live with pain ... I have.

On July 25, 1982, mother was back in the hospital with blood clots in her legs and lungs combined with a heart attack. She also had a broken leg from a fall; it was necessary to put two pins in the leg because the bone was so shattered. Mother also bruised a lung and kidney in the fall; and while she was in the hospital she suffered heart failure. She was sent to the University Hospital in Iowa City for two weeks.

After mother came home, I was the one who took care of her the most; many people did not feel that I would be able to do it because of my handicap. However, it was me or she would have to stay in the hospital because we did not have the money to hire someone to help us. It was also up to me to keep the house up, do the cooking and grocery shopping, and all other errands. Paula was suppose to help but she was too busy with her family and her husband's business. Many friends, family members, Public Health Nurse, and a homemaker helped out as much as they could. Rebecca Hayes also helped because she was a family friend.

During mother's recovery, it was necessary for Paula and I to go back to the doctor. Paula was having trouble with her sciatic nerve that ran through her hip and leg. The pain in my legs was spreading up into my back and lungs, making it difficult to care for mother at times. The doctor informed me that eventually my entire body would be in pain; I have arthritis so bad that I have the bones of a ninety-six year old woman and this is probably what causes the pain. I am not totally sure about this however. 1984 was to bring more bad luck. In January, I fell and broke my right arm, this was the one time it really was from a fall but the hospital did not believe me. Everyone in the emergency kept asking me if I was sure the injury was from a fall. I had to hold my arm above my heart for forty-eight hours so that I wouldn't form blood clots because the break was so severe. Unfortunately it was my right arm which is suppose to be my "good" arm and this made life quite interesting. On May 25, mother was air - lifted to Iowa City again with another heart attack and more blood clots. In September, one day after we officially closed the store, mother fell and broke her wrist but it never properly healed. Mother is also totally disabled now.

Over the years since I left, mother has had numerous health problems. She too had two open heart surgeries but she never felt well afterwards. I felt sorry for her but I could never had went back to take care of her because of my own failing health. Yes it has been a long struggle, but through it all came stronger faith and richer love. Mother died after we had a reconciliation and forgave each other for the past, on January 12, 2003.

CHAPTER 11: THE MIRACLES OF GOD

I remember when I was younger it was hard for me to go to the Sunday School classes at my church. With my braces having a strap on the back to keep my legs together and straight, it made getting up and down the steps difficult. When I did go, the teachers and minister would watch me to make sure I got there alright. Another problem I had in church was taking communion because the cup was too small for me. Elda, a good friend of mine whom I sat with at church helped me with communion; before I left the church when I left Ottumwa, we poured my communion in a cup that was easier for me to handle.

On occasion, I rode home from church with Elda and we attended many of the church functions together. Every year Elda would ask me to attend the Mother/Daughter banquet with her, Elda didn't have any children of her own. Occasionally the two of us would talk about our beliefs. I found that we both had the same concepts on how God works and why he does what he does with our lives.

I always felt that God wanted me to do whatever possible for the disabled, care for my family, go through the struggles I have gone through and overcome everything and make a life for myself. Also, Elda and I shared the same opinion that God had/has an assignment for each of us while on Earth. When I left home, Elda came to see me a few times, and Mary and I tried to visit her whenever we went to Ottumwa; but I always knew that Elda was close to my family and I didn't want her to get hurt. Even though there was an age gap between us, the two of us got along pretty well. Elda passed away in 1992.

Many people in our church feel very close to my family. I remember that when we were baptized, many of the ladies helped us in our preparations. These people are still very close to us even though we do not attend church on a regular basis.

During my parent's illness, I found out that many people were deeply concerned about the whole family. I realized that they were praying for my parents on a daily basis, but in the early80's I was told that I was also included in those prayers; by this time everyone was starting to see a change that NOONE liked. I was more withdrawn and depressed. This made me realize that the church was closer to us than I had thought.

The minister tried to get me to talk about what was bothering me, but that was just not my way. He knew that I had tried suicide and things were not the best for me at home, but I just would not open up. Our church was having services out of town at other churches and I would ride with his family, but still I did not talk about anything.

Although I am no longer able to attend church, I strongly believe in God. If it had not been for the work of God's powers, I would not be here to write this book. Everyday we hear about the things people do wrong; but very seldom do we hear about the work of God.

Today in many of the adult church classes, you will find them talking about the concerns and

problems of the world (such as abortion), instead of what God accomplished while on the face of the Earth. I sometimes wonder if maybe the church is so disturbed about the way things are, they forget about God. If this is true, then maybe it is time that we sit down and study our values of religion.

I am trying to discover what God has planned next for me. I know that writing this book was to be one of my major assignments. I also feel that he wants me to teach people about those who are handicapped. I truly believe that whatever he has me to do, it will involve the miracles of His work. It says in the Bible, "WHOEVER BELIEVETH IN ME SHALL NOT PERISH, BUT HAVE EVERLASTING LIFE." I feel that this statement is true. It is very important in our lives to really take each moment of each day and live it to its fullest; for this is the way God wanted us to do, for that is the way God did it while on Earth.

Like most people, I too have trouble telling others of the blessings He has given me. However, in order to help others find or let God into their lives, we need to share our experiences with Him, and this includes me. I feel that through my past experiences that I along with other people know the direction in which God has planned for them; and I feel that my destiny has been planned too. But I and many other people are uncertain of what steps to take to accomplish these assigned tasks. Maybe it is time we all stop to look around us, then and only then, can we truly be headed in the right direction that He planned for us.

With my Heavenly Father in mind, I feel that I can now inform people about the different tasks he has in store for the handicapped. Through my work, either this book and/or publicly speakingon behalf of the handicapped, I feel that I can educate the public by telling them of the differnt handicaps and how they effect people. I do nt quite understand why,but so manypeopl aeafraid and ashamed of the fact that there are those who are a little different from themselves. Anew public awareness is being made as more and more handicapped individuals are coming out into the public.

No longer are people afraid of the handicapped, because people can now see that the differences are really not that great. People are now able to see the handicapped as productive individuals, not individuals that one must feel sorry for or ashamed of. There isn't ridicule among people so much anymore, but there is a feeling of compassion as the handicapped are proving that they DO have a place in society. The phrase, "ALL MEN ARE CREATED EQUAL" now has meaning in the world that we live in. If we just remember this saying, I feel that each person has a chance in life to succeed. With God's help, maybe we as a society can get along with each other.

Through the years, I have noticed that society is beginning to accept the handicapped as people, not someone to put back in a corner or closet. I hope that as a society, we can learn to accept each other and NO one will be treated differently.

I was once asked by several college students how I felt attending college with non handicapped students. Many were surprised to hear me say that it really did not bother me. I had learned from some of the students and staff that they saw me as a hero. When I found this out, I asked them why they felt that way. Many of the same people told me that they did not know where I got all of my courage to handle the type of life my handicap and personal life caused, I told them it all went back to my theory that God is on my side.

I feel that it is through God, that I found the strength to return to college. Also, I hope that through my faith and courage, that I will be able to do anything I set my mind to.

I feel that faith has a valuable lesson for people, but there are many who are too stubborn to learn it. I have found that many people do not believe there is a God; and this makes me wonder how they think they got on Earth and how they get through daily life.

Because I chose to share my intimate love with someone of the same sex, it is not "morally " right for me to attend church. Some of our family and friends are still ashamed of us while others give us their love and support. Marie, a teacher who I will talk about later in the book, and I were talking one day about the way I chose to live; she told me that there was so little love in this world at times, she couldn't see anything wrong with the way I lived. I told her thank you for her understanding and support. I admit that people can't understand the way I feel, but as Marie told me. "As long as you are happy and well Deb, that's all that really matters. I feel that I don't have to worry so much about you this way. "

Dear Heavenly Father,

You are the light for us all and many you must call. But
 if it is you will, I will never sit still. So until the end,
 let me tell of the message that you send. And then
 Lord, you will find, I too have a feeling of peace in
 my mind.

Amen

CHAPTER 12: BITS AND PIECES
FROM MY LIFE

If we should meet along the way, it makes no difference
of the place, we should not feel dismay, for we will
all be in God's grace.

Deb

U sually we find people out on their own once they become "of
age;" but I was thirty-three before I finally got out on my own.
In 1974 just before I left college, my father filled out an application for
me to receive Supplemental Security Income (SSI), which was forty-nine
dollars a month. At the same time, Vocational Rehabilitation was arranging
for me to work at the Public Library. However, since my application for
SSI was approved, I was not able to take the job. The SSI program had/
has many rules for the participants, such as the blind, disabled and/or
elderly, to follow. For an example they must keep track of their money
very carefully. If another agency, such as heating assistance or low-income
housing assistance, helps a SSI participant, they must report this assistance
right away to the Social Security Administration, and many times this will
affect their monthly checks. Because I receive Social Security and SSI
both I do not have to report my assistance quite as much.

I feel that life is the main theme of this book. What it is, what can
happen to someone during life, and what you can do to live life to its
fullest. Life is like this fast paced world of ours – you learn to adapt to
meet your needs in order to survive.

I reached my education goal in 1993 when I received a Bachelor's of Art degree in English from the University of Iowa. After trying for many months after graduating to get a job, I realized that I would not be able to get a job. Harley and I were talking after I came to this realization, he told me he knew I would never be able to get a job but I was able to get an education and out of a bad situation; I will always respect him for telling me this and giving me moral support when it was needed. However, there are still times when I still want a job.

As the years of my life goes by, I realize that I will not be able to experience the type of life that a "normal" person does. I will always have an empty feeling in my heart when it comes to supporting myself and not living on government programs. During the rest of my life I hope to open many more doors of opportunity for the handicapped.

After I realized the severity of my CP, I understood the importance of making the public more aware of the handicapped and accepting them, along with fighting for accessibility of public facilities would always be my assignment while on Earth. I first realized this when I was to be the first severely handicapped student to be mainstreamed into the "regular" school system in my area; there had been a few mildly handicapped students mainstreamed before me. This main streaming was to be considered as an experiment that once started there would be no turning back; which was no easy task on my part; thus there was a lot of pressure on me to succeed when I started the main streaming program. I knew from the beginning that I had to make it or I would be considered a failure.

As an individual I want to be as independent as possible; in the late 90's I started to need more and more help. Today, I depend on that help so I can stay out of a nursing home or institution. Not exactly the independent life I had hoped for. This may sound unusual to you the reader, but I want to go out and do as much as I can as long as I possibly can. I feel that this will help me feel as if I am accepted in society.

Dreams and goals are set by each of us as individuals, but for some it takes a little longer to achieve them. Through the years I have seen so much deterioration in the form of economic, social and physical conditions of society as a whole; it makes me wonder if achieving anything in life is worthwhile. As a person I have no guarantee of what kind of life I can expect or what the future holds for me. I do know however that I must push myself more and more daily to keep surviving in daily life. I realize that I must stop and think before I move and this is still very frustrating at times. I face each daily struggle as another hurdle that has been jumped for victory to be made.

Sometimes I find myself wondering as I'm laying in bed at night and can't sleep, if life is really worth it. Many people, including myself are faced with an everyday struggle of just getting up and facing the routine of daily life. I often wonder if any of the struggle is worthwhile. I feel that each of us is going through some type of trip while fighting to survive in this world, but as I was once told, for some of us the trip is much further and harder than it is for others.

A friend once told me that he admired me for my perseverance. At the time I thought he was just being nice, but in reality, he was telling me that he could not understand where I got all of my determination and willpower to keep fighting each day just to survive. I reminded him that it was God who gave me the strength to fight and it certainly wasn't just me doing the fighting because there were many times I would have given up.

One day while at the doctor's office in Ottumwa, I was trying to make it easier for the nurse who was working with me; as she worked with me, she told me it was alright for her to have to work a little harder with me than she did the other patients. She also told me she doubted if she could do as well as I did just going through the everyday battles of everyday life. This made me stop and think about rather being "normal," by this I mean being able to move your body without any difficulties, is so easy after all. Yes sometimes just living everyday is a constant battle when you are trapped inside. Your mind may work well, but your body can't In order to survive all of this, it takes a lot of perseverance and determination, but unlike a normal person, I have to make up my mind ahead of time to WIN my share of battles.

When ever I go out to eat with friends, I try to order something simple, like Chicken Nuggets instead of a Big Mac, so that I would not embarrass them or make a mess all over. There are times when I will feel at ease and order anything I want. The ordering something simple was mainly so that the people around me would not get upset or embarrassed by the way I eat. Many handicapped people, including myself, knows what it is like to be ridiculed because they are different.

Maybe this is why life is so strange to me. It makes me realize that each and every one of us, whether we have a noticeable handicap or not, must make our life count as much as possible. I hope that other people can feel the same way that I do. During each individual's trip through life, the question that most commonly comes to mind, "is life worth it?" My answer to this question is yes, but only if you can make life and all of its struggles worth the ups and downs, can you have a feeling of self worth. This is what is required in each of us to truly be a person.

As I worked on this book, many memories went through my mind that I did not know how to express in writing. I did not realize all of the events I did remember. Most people don't think about their memories, but it was those same memories that made writing my book possible.

Memories of my life are in this book. I have made many mistakes in my life and at the same time I have accomplished things no one thought would be possible; however I am not totally ashamed of myself. Some of these mistakes hurt my family as well as myself. I thought my family was happy for me when I returned to college, but I soon found out that they considered me as a bitch, retarded, and wasting my time and taxpayers money. I could never please my family no matter how hard I tried.

At various times in my life, I have asked a few people what it is like to be "normal" but so far I have not gotten an answer. Everyone tells me that they can't answer my question because they do not know what it feels like being trapped in my body. That is really what being handicapped is, being trapped and limited on what your body can do.

Many people have given their description on how they feel that I have overcome the obstacles of
society. While at the same time a few of my friends did not feel that they could write about working with me. It was their opinion that watching me and helping me was just a part of the normal process of living. I have been told by many that they admire me for my determination, courage and perseverance, but to me this was also just a part of everyday living.

These words from the song, THE IMPOSSIBLE DREAM, express some of my feelings that I have inside. "IF ONE MAN TATTERED AND TORN WITH SCARS, CAN FIGHT WITH HIS LAST OUNCE OF COURAGE TO REACH THE UNREACHABLE STAR." Then I think that each and every one of must do this. So please try to remember this in everything you do in life, and I know this world will be a better place for all of us to live in. So pour out your love and wait with me to see what happens in this world of ours.

In my early years, the handicapped were kept at home. Therefor, fear and shame are two emotions that would accompany me and other handicapped people throughout life. Fear is present in my life because of the abuse I went through and because I do not know how people will react from me. From the ages of eight to thirty-three, I went through every type of abuse there is; if I did not cooperate with what was being done to me by multiple men, the abuse would worsen. Not many girls would be drugged because they did not want sexual abuse to happen every night to them, however I was given drugs, beaten, or tied up for not cooperating.

Shame is a part of me because of my handicap. I have experienced rejection, ridicule and both physical and mental abuse because I am different. An example of my shame is being afraid to eat in front of strangers. My CP makes it difficult for me to eat without being ashamed to ask for help. Places with buffets are nice to eat at, but I have to have someone get the food as well as cutting it for me; as a person who is almost fifty, this is VERY embarrassing. No matter what your age, try to put yourself in my shoes and I think you will understand my feelings.

It has been said that I was/am withdrawn and insecure at times. I think these feelings are such an important part of me because I never knew/know how people were/are going to react towards me, so I am not always sure if I am passing the scrutiny of society. I am that focused on how people will react to me and it bothers my friends and helpers that I let other peoples' acceptance of me rule my life. Also, I was afraid because I did not know who, when or why I would be abused.

This was never more true than my time in the "main streaming experiment." During my years attending the regular school system, many of my teachers fought with the school board over rather I needed to be placed in the special education classes or not. I did not know of this matter until my senior year of high school when I was working on an outside assignment for one of my classes. This assignment was an in depth look at how the school system dealt with the different types of handicapped students. At first it was necessary for many of these handicapped students that were a part of the main streaming program to be placed into the special education classes while the teachers were instructed on how to cope with the situation. I know many of the teachers had to learn how to cope and work with me while I was in their class because they were not given any advanced training or warning before I started main streaming.

Many of the handicapped can not make very much progress in school because of their handicap; because it is mandatory for all students to have a chance to an education, the teachers would instruct them as much as possible. It was during an interview with one of the special education teachers for my assignment that I learned about the constant battle with the school board.

As the years go by, I find that society is beginning to accept the handicapped more. I feel this was partially due to the main streaming program.

Near the end of the store business people entered the store and was able to carry on a conversation with me without being afraid of me. Today's society seems to accept the handicapped better than yesterday's society, partially because of the fact there is more education about the

67

many handicaps and partially because the handicapped are out in public more. With this being true, the handicapped can come out of their corners of hiding and shed their feelings of shame.

Just like the song MEMORIES, everything in this book is through the memories and experiences of my life. In some ways, I have lived a sheltered life, while at the same time, I had to overcome many obstacles to be able to survive in the world. I hope that each and every person on Earth can have both good and bad memories because this is what shapes us as individuals. It takes a few bad memories for a person to learn through their mistakes. The good memories gives a person hope for a better tomorrow. A better tomorrow .... I wonder if there is such a thing. Life can throw some pretty hard blows, I know because I have had a few.

Dear God,

Place me into the world to work toward my goals
through your help and my courage. But most of all,
let Your eternal love guide me through my work. In
Your Name I pray.

Amen

CHAPTER 13: THE HANDICAPPED ADULT GROUP

Have you ever wondered what happens to the handicapped after they become of age? For many it is a life of idleness. In 1976 the local Cerebral Palsy Association and I tried forming a group that would try to help alleviate the idleness of the handicapped by providing a recreational activity for them once a month.

The work that was involved in setting up these activities was sometimes very frustrating; but I hoped from every effort that I put into the group, someone was able to receive something from it. I found that many of the individuals and their families were ashamed of the fact that there was/is such a thing as a physical or mental handicap. This is due to the fact that society has enforced and reinforced this feeling.

Once you are ashamed or embarrassed by someone who is handicapped, it seems as if you always feel that way.

The main purpose of the group was to provide a recreational program for those who otherwise did not have the chance to get out and enjoy themselves otherwise. Another purpose of the group was to talk over some of the everyday problems that was being faced by the handicapped members. Some of those problems could be solved as a group while it was necessary for the Government or Legislation to work out others.

The group was not aimed at involving the handicapped it also served the purpose of integrating the non-handicapped population as helpers with the group. I felt that this was necessary in order for the handicapped to be accepted. There is a song titled, NO MAN IS AN ISLAND, that I feel/felt fit(s) each and every one of us. I hope that in the present and the future, that not one person is frowned upon because he/she is handicapped.

There was a lot of work connected with the group. Not only was I involved with group activities, but I was a board member of the local Cerebral Palsy Association, which meant that I had to attend the monthly meetings. I also was required to attend as many State meetings as possible, and this involved traveling and gathering my needed information. Also there was a lot of literature that dealt with important issues that was connected in some way to the group members, that had to be ordered, read and a report presented to group members; however, most of the group did not understand or comprehend what was being talked about. I often found that I needed to set aside a day every once in awhile just to read and deal with the incoming material. I did not mind doing this if I felt that the group and their families appreciated the information I was gathering and distributing to the group.

All in all, the group usually kept me busy. My family was very angry at times how busy I was, and if I had enjoyed our outings, my family let me know of their disapproval in front of my co-chairman. She witnessed a lot of verbal and emotional abuse that was being done to me and I felt very sorry for her. I felt the group was successful when I was able to help someone on their way to leading a "normal" productive life. Not only was I trying to help the members of the group but I was trying to help myself at the same time. It was unusual for a group leader to feel this way, but with the work I was doing, this seemed to be true.

Due to the lack of interest and my increased family responsibilities, the group was discontinued on September 26, 1977. I felt this was the best decision considering all the efforts and frustrations I was facing at the time. To me the poor attendance, I and my co-leader were often the only ones that showed up, it was best not to keep the group in existence.

I thought the handicapped were being accepted by most people until a few years ago when I read a letter written in a Dear Abby column. There was a comment made by a bystander about where the handicapped should sit when eating out in public. It made me wonder how many people are still afraid of the handicapped. The writer felt that the handicapped should be made to sit in the back of the restaurant while eating. In my opinion this is segregation because every person should have a freedom of choice on where he wants to sit. I feel that people cannot accept us if they are not around the situation in order to learn to handle it. I really am not that much different from everyone else, but there are some things that I still need help with and this will always be the case for me.

Feelings are another important part of a person's life. Not only do we have them, but it is vitally important that we can express them when we need to. On occasion I find this very hard to do. All during my life I have been told by some that you keep your feelings inside, and at the same time, others have told me that it was okay to express my feelings. At times these concepts have kept me confused about expressing my feelings. However for the handicapped it is very difficult for them to express their feelings.

> AS WE CROSS DUSTY ROADS,
> LET US FIND SOMEONE TO SHARE THE LOADS.
> WHEN WE FIND THAT PERSON,
> WE MUST REMEMBER THAT IT IS OUR GIFT
>   FROM HEAVEN.
> SO GO FAR MY FRIEND.
> USE THE TREASURED GIFT GOD HAS SENT.
> WE MUST GET THE MESSAGE THAT IS MEANT.
> OR WE ALL WILL LOSE IN THE VERY END.

> Deb

CHAPTER 14: SPECIAL PEOPLE AND OTHER THINGS

FRIENDS

There are people who are always there. Someone who
    has extra time to care.
Never lose them you see or else you must concede. They
    really do help in time of need.

Deb

Having a lot of friends my own age is one of life's pleasures that I missed out on. True I do have a lot of friends, but most of them are older than I am. I could never really communicate with people my own age because many of them were either afraid of me or thought I was contagious. It took me a long time to understand why people were/are afraid of me. Once I finally understood, I wanted to help people see that inside I was just like them.

Many of my fellow classmates told me this the week before we graduated from high school. They believed if they touched me or got too close tp me, they would automatically get Cerebral Palsy; little did they know that I was afraid of them for a long time. I didn't understand why I wasn't or couldn't be like them. I can now laugh about it and understand where they got their beliefs when I think of the slogan about cerebral palsy, which goes "it strikes like lightning every fifty-three seconds." The fear that people had/have of this slogan made/makes me realize the need to educate about the different handicaps and the feeling that accompanying those dealing with the different handicaps.

Every three years I would participate in the local telethon for CP, many of my friends from school would see me and be full of questions the next day. I remember that many would ask me about being on the stage with the actors and actresses that was helping to raise the money, and others would come up and ask me if the participants that was on the stage with me were real. I remember telling a lot of them if they went over to meet the students at Smith- Warren, they would see how real the other participants.

One day as a class project we went to Smith-Warren and that is when my fellow classmates started to accept me. While they were taking the tour, I was going through my therapy session and they had the chance to see what I did while they were in gym. After we returned to class, many asked me if the treatments that they had observed me doing hurt, I told them no but it was necessary for me to do in order to get through daily life. Many expressed that they didn't know if they could endure my life, I told them anything was possible once you set your mind to it. Granted many eyes were opened that day but not all of the peer ridicule stopped.

Rhonda Little, who was the Public Health Nurse and a friend of mine up until her death, had these thought about me she wanted to share.

"I first saw Debbie when she came home from the hospital after her birth. Most babies come home in three days but Debbie had to stay for a longer stay due to her handicapping condition. After each visit that I made as a nurse to see Debbie and her family, I remember coming home and bragging about her eyes and how cute she was. Also, I remember seeing her at the Smith-Warren School when I did volunteer work and helped with the parties."

"I remember helping with the 1957 telethon for Cerebral Palsy, Debbie was a part of it even though she couldn't do very much yet. Since then, I have worked as a chairman on all of the telethons. Through the years of telethons, I became better acquainted with Debbie, and for many of us, Debbie was the inspiration we needed when things were going bad for us. Debbie is a walking quadriplegic, and each activity that she participates in takes three times as much energy for Debbie than it does for most of us. Although Debbie walks, she doesn't realize that she is using all of her strength, that's the way life is for her. "

"Throughout the 1977 telethon, Debbie helped me and the other workers just by being there. She was our inspiration and an example of the clients we helped. Had it not been for Debbie and the other clients, many of us would have given up. Debbie told us to cheer up because at least we had a little more money to help our CP clients, and she was right! Since then we talk to each other, go out together, and share a strong and understanding relationship. I look at Debbie and feel very proud that I know her."

In 1982, Rhonda passed away. She ended up spending her last years fighting Leukemia and Cancer. A few months before Rhonda died, she had loaned us a shampoo stand to make it easier for Rebecca to wash mother's hair while she was in a wheelchair. I was going to return this to Carl, but he said Rhonda had wanted me to keep it. The words from Kenny Nolan's song, LOVE'S GROWN DEEP is how both Rhonda and Carl felt about our relationship." Later in life other friends would also become a part of me.

> SOMEWHERE BACK IN TIME. YOU BECAME A
> FRIEND OF MINE. DAYBY DAY, WE GREW
> A LITTLE CLOSER. YOU'RE MY SPIRIT TO
> BE STRONG, A FRIENDWHEN THINGS GO
> WRONG. SO I'VE WRITTEN DOWN THESE
> WORDS TO LET YOUKNOW. LOVE'S GROWN
> DEEP IN THE HEART OF ME, YOU'VE
> BECAME A PART OF ME!

Other people have shared some thoughts with me. The first is my Grandmother on my father's side. She passed away in December, 1989.

"Well Debbie, you asked me to write what you meant to Grandpa and me. This is pretty hard for me to do because you certainly meant a lot to both of us."

"I very well remember the night you were born. Your father came and tapped on the window about two or three o'clock in the morning. He told us that your mother and he had a baby girl but they were very much afraid that you would not live long because you were badly injured at birth. Believe me, we prayed for you and your mother. When we were allowed to visit, we came to the hospital to see you. The nurse wheeled up the prettiest little baby with a great big lot of black curls; the nurse had brushed them into ringlets a put a yellow bow on top. Grandpa said, "that baby is going to stay here, we aren't going to lose her." He thought such a pretty fat little baby just had to be alright."

"When you were going to Iowa City for your treatments or therapy or whatever it was called, we were hopeful for you. When you were wearing those heavy braces, we prayed for the time to get rid of them. Also, it did bother Grandpa to see you wear the weights on your arms."

"We were always proud of your progress in school. I was so sorry to see you quit college, but I knew you were old enough to make up your mind and knew how you felt better than I did."

"When I see how well you are doing and all the things you do, I am so thankful you are able to do what you do."

"Well Debbie, I know this isn't much, but I can say in a few words to the question, "What did I mean to you?" I can say that I did know that you were and always would be very dear to us."

The following lines are from Nina Gray, one of my caseworkers from the late 70's until I left Ottumwa in 1987.

" I first became acquainted with Debbie in 1977 when I requested help from the Cerebral Palsy funds for a helmet for another client. At the time Debbie's father, Peter, handled the funding in Wapello County. I was instantly taken with Deb — an attractive young woman who, although suffering from cerebral palsy herself, was more interested in the problems of others than herself."

"Since birth Deborah has had Cerebral Palsy. Though I was not acquainted with her in her early years, she had and has determination. She attended regular classes in school and the Ottumwa Heights College. This was no easy feat — books to carry, steps to climb, crowded hallways — Yet Deb managed."

"For years she has assisted her parents in their grocery store, frequently being the only one in attendance. She also manages a small second hand shop to sell and display her hand made woven mats and other craft items"

"Deborah's great love and feeling of responsibility for her parents is to be commended. During these past few years, Deb has been the "mainstream" of the family when her parents were hospitalized and during recovery periods. Always without a complaint, Deb "carried" her load and then some. She has desired to live independently and has worked toward this goal. It seems as if God is not ready for this because she and her parents remain interdependent."

Nina shared these comments long before I left home, and she shared them from her heart as she worked with me. As she once said, it was rare that I asked for help.

Christmas always was special to me for the fact it is our Savior's birth. It was a time to rejoice in the fact that God gave us his only Son to save us from whatever wrong there would be in our lives. It also is a time when the love we have for others has the chance to be truly shown. Also it is a day we set aside to spend with family and/or friends. May we all remember this so there can be Peace on Earth, Goodwill towards men.

I would tolerate the holidays the best I could, but because I was/am allergic to the scents of Christmas, I was usually sick with bronchitis. When I think of Christmas, I think of the birth of Jesus. However the Christmas of 1975 was special because Paula surprised us all by giving birth to a son; no one including Paula, knew that she was pregnant. Alan, my nephew, was a pleasant surprise who weighed seven pounds, six and a half ounces when he was born.

Alan was too young to know all of the love that surrounded him that Christmas day. For a while, I looked forward to spending the holidays with him, but as he grew older that was to change too. Even though there was a new addition to the family that year, one could sense the fake love that was in the house. Each time we got together as a family, I prayed that things would change, but because of the hate and abuse, I knew it wouldn't happen.

At Christmas time we see various organizations helping the needy and less fortunate. While in Ottumwa, I would go to the Salvation Army for food baskets at holiday time; in Iowa City, I have received help from Project Holiday. I have a problem with this when I see people driving up in expensive cars and wearing fancy clothes to receive help when they really don't need the help. It really bothers me to see the agencies that offer help for the needy get taken advantage of.

> Christ was born today.
> His Love surrounds us all.
> Raise up your troubles to him.
> Instantly you will feel him by your side.
> Sing to rejoice him.
> Thank you Lord for caring for us.
> Mary was his mother.
> Angels are everywhere.
> Savior, we adore Thee.

Deb

CHAPTER 15: INDIAN HILLS COMMUNITY COLLEGE

On November 18, 1986, I returned to college to pursue a degree in Library Science which the job proved to be too much for me. Then it was to be Social Work but I ended up getting a Bachelor's of Art degree in English. My previous college expenses, 1973 - 1974, were paid for by the local Cerebral Palsy Association and Vocational Rehabilitation, when I returned to college, my expenses were paid through Vocational Rehabilitation and Federal Grants. My goal upon returning to college was to open new doors for myself.

I was in fairly good health when I started classes, but as time went on, my strength, energy and enthusiasm was not there anymore. This worried everyone that was working with me; especially Marie, who was one of my teachers, and Joe who was my Vocational Rehabilitation counselor. I had not told anyone at the college about the abuse I was going through on top of caring and supporting my family while I was also trying to keep up my studies.

One day when Marie and I were finished with discussing my research paper, she asked me, "What's wrong Deb? I notice a fast change in you and your health and I am having a lot of trouble believing that it's just pressure from school. What is happening with you? I've talked to Joe and he told me he's worried too." I told her I couldn't talk about it and everything would be okay.

But Marie wouldn't accept this and said I was not moving until I told her what was wrong. I kept trying to convince her that it would be okay, but she just wouldn't accept my answer. She kept trying to get me to talk to her about whatever it was that was bothering me so that she could try to help. So I finally talked until it was time for class to begin. After class, Marie joined me for lunch. She told me that legally she was obligated to report the abuse, but she was going to try to help me get out instead.

Because we had talked on a day that I had my evening class and Marie was staying late to work on a play she would be presenting in March, she joined me for supper. I thought she was going to stroke out when she saw that the rest of my lunch was my supper. Her first question was, "will you be eating more when you get home?" I told her no and not to worry about it. She then wanted to buy me a meal or get food for me to take home but I told her we would be alright and I was just making food stretch more because of the holidays coming up. That was the wrong words to say to Marie because she wanted more information about my family.

I then explained to her that both parents were ill and disabled and they had a lot of back bills to pay. I was trying to do as much as I could but the doctor wanted me to get out before it killed me, so toward the end-of-the month and holidays we made our food go further. She didn't like the sound of this but knew that it would be best not to push the issue.

About this time, I was starting to trust and feeling close to Marie, and I found out from another teacher that she was starting to feel very close to me. In reality, this is why I was able to start trusting and confiding in her. I was finally able to tell someone what was happening to me as an adult. Believe me, Marie became more worried, concerned and scared for me as I finally started to talk about the abuse.

After trying suicide over the five week break from school, I was even more of a nervous wreck upon returning for the spring semester. I was going to Marie's play in March with Paula, but the stress, abuse and pressure was getting to be way too much for me. After I made the mistake of telling Marie that I was planning another attempt to commit suicide, she called Joe at his office. I had told Marie that I wouldn't be coming back to classes the next week, she asked me why, and like an idiot I told her. She did not let me out of her sight until Joe got there. Both of them sensed that I was close to the breaking point. Joe came to Marie's office and we talked. Joe asked my permission to talk to my family about the situation and he wanted to talk to them about moving me into the dorm so I could get used to it before moving me to Iowa City. Joe was even more frustrated when they laughed at him and wouldn't listen to anything he had to say. After Joe left, Mother started calling me "a thing or a piece of trash" and that really hurt. Mother wasn't going to let me go to class the next day but father reminded her that if I wasn't there, Joe would be back in the afternoon. They were afraid of him, but Joe was not afraid of them, he let my parents know that he meant business.

The play was at this same time. Joe saw Paula and I there but he was told by Paula to get away. Joe made a special point to be at Marie's office on Monday. He could tell at the play, I had been punished and was hurting. His wife was from DHS and was ready to help Joe in any way possible.

The day after Joe's visit, Marie asked me how things went. When I was telling her, Joe walked into her office and asked what happened after he left. I told them both at the same time and they both became more worried and concerned. At one point Marie tried to get me to go to the Crisis Center, but I was even too scared to do this. Both of them kept worrying until I got out.

I tried to leave but I kept getting more scared. Marie and I even changed my address with Social Security one time, but later that day I sensed something was wrong and cancelled the change. When I got home that night my uneasiness was confirmed when my parents told me about the Social Security office calling to let them know I had tried to change my address. I was severely punished and the bruises were very noticeable to Marie the next day; she had commented on the fact that I was so scared and beaten it was like I was back at square one. I wanted out but I was too afraid to try again for a while.

Both Marie and Joe noticed my increased fear, lack of sleep, and the fact I wasn't eating very much, if at all, so they tried to get me to talk to them or someone else and wanted me to LEAVE soon. Because my parents were mad and more abusive towards me since Joe had talked to my family, I did not want either of them to get hurt; but they both kept assuring me that they could protect themselves and me too. It took a long time before I got the courage to leave, but when I did get brave enough, Marie was there for me. Two weeks before I left my family Alan, my twelve year old nephew, had taken a butcher knife and pointed it at my forehead between my eyes; the next day he was trying to poke my eyes out with a pair of scissors. The fear of being hurt or killed was so intense I got to the point where it I wasn't eating or sleeping and this worried Marie even more as she watched me going downhill even faster.

On the day I told Marie about my nephew she asked me when I was going to get strong enough to leave. I told her without any hesitation, "in two weeks. Will you still help me?" She said, "YES, but why are you waiting that long." I explained that Joe needed that long to arrange for Vocational Rehabilitation to pay for my room and meal ticket for the semester; he too told her that later in the day and said he wanted everything to fall in place so I would start looking better.

When moving week came, the day before I left, Marie read the note I was leaving in the mailbox the next day before coming to school. She was waiting in her office for me the next day. She asked me how I was doing, I told her scared and nervous; she then told me that was natural but everything would be okay. The two of us became closer that day and she stuck by me the entire time.

After lunch that day my teacher told me I had a note from Marie, this surprised me as we had just seen each other. I asked permission to go to see her and find out what was wrong. She told me to see Joe after class. I asked her if there was a problem and if I had to go home. Marie told me there was a problem, I would not be going home and to be sure to see Joe. I went to see Joe but he was checking with some other staff people about the problem; he told the kitchen staff to keep me there. They gave me a coke to drink and told me to wait for Joe. A little later he came back and told me that my father and sister called him and they wanted to see me right now. We talked about it and decided if the meeting did take place he was going to be there the whole time and at the school and not at home. Joe then called father back to let him no the rules for the meeting but they refused the offer.

Later father called Joe again and threatened a lawsuit against everyone including me. Joe told him to go ahead but he wouldn't win. This made father furious so he went to see Harley. Harley told him to forget it; then he became very brave and said to his brother, "you don't love Deb, you only want her for her money. Also, Deb is better off now." I was very surprised when Harley told me this in later years. Paula was also attending school here, so she thought she could get any information she wanted. When she asked for my room number and my class schedule, the Dean called Joe to let him know. Joe reinforced the rule that NOBODY was to get any information about me; he then came to see Marie and I to warn us there was new trouble stirring. Back in hiding I went and Paula was mad so she quit school.

Since I had very little when I left, Marie and Bev, another teacher helped me with money, clothes, groceries and items for my room. They were joined by many of the other staff members and students to get me settled in. Rebecca and Sharon, a close friend who chose to support me instead of my family, helped as much as they could. I called Sharon just before Thanksgiving to let her know I was okay and that I would be going to the Crisis Center for Thanksgiving weekend. The first words out of her mouth were, "where in the hell are you and where in the hell have you been?" I told her why the delay in calling so she calmed down. She then asked me if I was alright and what I needed and told me not to be afraid to tell her the truth. The next day she was out to see me and let me know that she would bring me Thanksgiving dinner to the center. When she came, she became worried because medically I wasn't doing very well. I told her I had seen a doctor and everything would be okay.

The week after Thanksgiving, I saw a cousin and her mother while I was waiting for class. They asked if I needed anything, I told them and they brought it to me. My aunt asked me where I would be for the holidays and I told them the Crisis Center but they COULD NOT tell my family that. Big mistake because my cousin called me Christmas day and wanted to come get me. I reminded her I couldn't come because my parents, sister and her family would be there. About then Grandma got on the phone and asked me the same thing, I said no. later that evening father was banging on the door at the center wanting in, but the staff had been called and they came and sent him away.

The holidays were rough for me but I got through them even with the complications of excessive bleeding from my monthly cycle. Bev, Sharon, and Rebecca took turns seeing and calling me; Marie had planned on coming to see me but her daughter was at home very sick; but Marie did call me when she could.

My stay at the center was unique because there was no heat, which was one of the reasons I couldn't hide in the dorm. Upon returning to school and the dorm where there was heat, I became very ill. I had so much infection in me that I was dizzy and "fading out, which was later diagnosed as petite mal seizures," a lot and I finally ended up going to the doctor after two weeks of being sick. Marie started to get worried when I wasn't back by lunch time. I got back five minutes before my first class, I had left my books in Marie's office so she would know that I returned okay. She was in her office talking to another student when I stopped by to get my books, but she stopped talking to find out what the doctor said. I told her that I was full of infection and that an antibiotic would be delivered later. Her next question was what about lunch, I told her there wasn't enough time but I would grab something to drink.

My last class for the day was with Marie, she knew I wasn't up to it so she didn't ask me to participate in reading that day. After class she asked me if I wanted to wait till supper time in her office, I told her that I wasn't hungry and was going to my room. This did not make her happy because she knew I hadn't eaten at noon either. After play rehearsal that night there was a knock on my door. I opened it to find Marie there holding a bowl of hot soup, but after looking at me, she knew I wasn't going to eat because I was getting sicker.

I told her I would be feeling better by Monday; I had forgot that Marie would be in every day of the weekend working on the play. During her breaks on Friday and Saturday, Marie was over checking on me. On Sunday I was feeling better so Marie asked me to join her in her office while she waited for her husband and daughters to come. When her family came I told her I would see her the next day and she politely informed me that she was walking me back to my room, her family had brought supper for all of us but I didn't find that out until we got to my room. I offered to go to the kitchen or lounge so that we could all eat together but Marie said no; I'm going to set yours up, you're going to eat and take your pill and go to sleep for awhile. I told you she was a typical mother hen. I asked where they were going to sit and she told me they would eat when they got home and she wanted me to rest.

I waited until lunch time to go over the next day. Marie came in as I was about to sit down while the kitchen staff was getting ready to cut my meat. Marie told them she would cut it as soon as she got her lunch. When she got to the table I told her she was to overprotective. She told me she knew that but that was part of her job and our friendship. She asked me if I was feeling any better, I told her yes but I wished I wouldn't sleep so much; she told me until all of the infection cleared up, I would sleep a lot. I was on an antibiotic for over a month.

Spring break was coming up and Marie asked me what I would be doing. I told her Joe was sending me for an evaluation at a group home in Des Moines. If I qualified, he was going to have me go there for college instead of Iowa City. I was at the facility for two hours and they had already determined that the place was inappropriate for me. They called and made the arrangements for me to return to Ottumwa the next day. I called Bev to let her know I was coming home a day early. While I was in Des Moines, I purchased a dress to wear to graduation.

After spring break Joe and I had to hurry and register me for classes at the University of Iowa. My application was processed fast and I was accepted for the summer term. This was a relief because none of us had to figure out what to do with me for the summer.

Marie was unable to attend my graduation because she had another commitment. On graduation day, I put my dress on so the two of us could have our picture taken together. Afterwards Marie told me she wished that had let me show her the dress so she could have made some alternations to it, I reminded her that I had tried to do so but she was pretty busy at the time. She then told me to make sure she was with me before I purchased any more clothes. I told her okay.

As a graduation present, Marie told me that she wanted to be the one to take me to Iowa City when I moved. Although Joe was a little uneasy about her taking me, it did make it easier in regards to how I was going to get there. Marie was very upset when she found out Joe had gone to The Lord's Cupboard, an agency that provides funds for people who are moving, to get gas money. He also told me that I was to give her fifty dollars for the trip. She took the money from Joe so that she could return it to him, but she would not take any money from me. She reminded me that I would need supplies for school.

After arriving in Iowa City, Marie took me out to eat and the grocery store while we waited for my room to be ready. Believe me Marie made sure I had enough groceries. Marie was very upset when she found out I would be spending the first two weeks in the dorm by myself. Now if you ask me, this is a typical mother hen reaction! I was told this but I was also told not to tell Marie. We both cried that night when it was time to say goodbye and for Marie to return to Ottumwa. Marie and Rebecca took turns coming up until I got settled in, it was very hard for all of us.

The day we came up we both met Ron and Jane Ron would be my Vocational Rehabilitation counselor, and Jane was the secretary for Services for People with Disabilities, SPD, where Diane and Jim would be my counselors. Jane was able to arrange for people to help keep me busy so Marie wouldn't worry so much, but she did anyway.

After summer school and work started, Marie went to see her parents in Wisconsin. But she made sure people were going to keep an eye on me before she went. Upon her return she tried to see me every week until it was time for her to go back to work. I think her family was glad to see school start so she would stay home. However, I was to call her at least once a week.

CHAPTER 16: LIFE IN BURGE HALL AT THE UNIVERSITY OF IOWA

In May of 1988, Burge Hall became my second home since I left home. I was enrolled for the summer semester at the University of Iowa. Children's Literature was a required course for Library Science so that was my class for the summer, I earned an A for the course. Mid way through the semester, there was a fire at the construction site outside my window. I lost three hundred dollars worth of personal belongings and food.

My family had found out how to get in contact with me through a cousin that worked for the college. They were constantly harassing me for things they needed or for money. I was dumb enough to send them money a couple of times and when Marie found out about it, she reminded me that I wasn't responsible for my family anymore. Even though we could no longer be around each other because of the abuse, I still loved them. Marie told me she understood that but I had to take care of me and not the world.

During the break between the summer and fall semester Ron helped me get a job at the Psychology Library and I worked very hard to learn the system that was used there. I also worked there for part of the fall and spring terms.

Life started to settle down once classes started in August. I was able to make friends with everyone except Mary.Mary was a non traditional student like myself but she tended to stay to herself which I felt was rare on a handicapped women's floor. If someone talked to her first, she would talk, but very seldom would she start a conversation. I wanted to know more about this stubborn person who tended to ignore everyone and wanted to be stranger to her dorm mates. I guess dorm life in Ottumwa taught me not to be a stranger.

One night after work I decided to confront Mary. If she needed a friend, I'd offer the hand of friendship. I was going to get this stubborn old broad to talk to me or know the reason why! I blocked her doorway with my wheelchair. She actually looked dumbfounded. She couldn't ignore that "Hi!" Mary was unhappy at my behavior but she finally talked to me. She was having trouble with her roommate and wanted nothing to do with anybody.

"Is there a reason you're ignoring me?" I asked.

"No" she said.

We introduced ourselves to each other. She had already been to super but we did talk for awhile with the promise to have super together the next day. We went to lunch and started talking while we ate. Mary noticed that I had several problems eating and asked if I ever thought about using weighted silverware. I told her I had tried it before but it didn't work. She came up with several suggestions but I had to tell her it had all been tried but nothing worked for me.

Mary has an emotional disability and three learning disabilities which makes life frustrating for her; she also has several medical problems. She did not want to get involved with anyone and devote all her time to studying. Boy did I ruin that! When people asked Mary why she got involved with me, I've heard her say that she recognized the suicidal signs that I was having; she was right but I was to ashamed to admit it.

Mary and I had a common connection in that we were both clients of Vocational Rehabilitation (VR) and Services for People with Disabilities (S P D). She was having trouble with V R and I was having trouble with SPD. Each of tried to convince the other that the problem department really wasn't so bad. The head of SPD was friends with my boss, so I could hardly go to her with problems at work. Mary didn't understand Ron. She didn't know how to talk to people and understood them less sometimes. This included Ron and NO ONE could help her because she didn't want to hear it!

Though she seemed to know people, she couldn't connect with them. Due to one of her learning disabilities, she frequently said the opposite of what she meant, this could prove to be embarrassing, frustrating, and uncomfortable for everyone. Even so, she had/has a heart of gold. She'd do anything for anyone. She was a Do-gooder, a "Buttinsky." We even got to the point where we called each other "buttinsky." This was another hang up of hers, she always wanted to help people even if they didn't know they needed help.

Several months after I became friends with Mary I asked her how she knew the effects of abuse. She indicated she had suffered from neglect and emotional abuse. I challenged her that it was the same thing and I learnt that you don't challenge Mary. That was a BIG MISTAKE! To cool off before we talked anymore she suggested we go to lunch.

We talked about the different types of abuse and how they effected people. We even had a fight because I thought emotional abuse was different. I found out how wrong I was. But after we talked, I knew that emotional abuse was just as bad. Mary had been abused emotionally by her family, so she knew some of the pain I was dealing with.

Mary gave me some examples of emotional abuse and neglect. She told me how she felt. We talked about the "false smile." We talked about how she was finally forced to get help under commitment and how "her Dr. Erickson" stuck it out with her until she was really ready to get help. She knew I was suicidal and said she'd help me find someone who could help me. Little did we know that we had to go through a rough summer in order for me to get help. If we had known the problems that awaited us, we probably would have done things differently. Mary made me promise that I would talk to someone before I did anything.

My fall term was rough. I had trouble with classes and had to drop several because the teachers wouldn't work with me and/or health reasons. I did not know it at this time, but I would be going to surgery soon. Lola, a Social Work student who was assigned to me through SPD, tried to help me with school, past abuse, health problems, work, and Doris, who was my boss; and she really did try, but because I saw her as an "authority figure" it didn't work out.

In October of 1988, I took myself over to the hospital in my electric wheelchair because I couldn't stop or slow down my monthly bleeding. The hospital wanted to keep me but I said "no" because no one knew where I was. Mary had gone home to Davenport for the weekend, and I didn't know how to get hold of Lola. I told them both within a forty-eight hour time frame that I had gone to the hospital and why, they were both worried. Mary had came by my room when she got back to Iowa City for me to go est with her and Dottie only to be told no because the hospital had told me to stay in bed for a few days.

After her and Dottie went to eat and Dottie was on her way home, Mary came in with something for me to eat and asked what happened. I told her the bleeding from my cycle was so bad I couldn't stand without blood going everywhere. The hospital let me come home but only if I stayed in bed for a few days. The only times I was out of bed was to eat, have something to drink, go to the bathroom and make the phone calls I had to make.

I called Doris to tel her that I wouldn't be in to work for two days because I was sick and spent part of the weekend in the hospital. When I returned to work we talked about what was going on before doing my duties that day. I worked that day but I also fell. Doris and I talked at the end of my shift and I told her that I thought it would be better if I quit until I was feeling better. She agreed and told me to keep her informed.

By Thanksgiving I had gone back to the hospital and knew that I would be having surgery; I was thirty-four, and felt like I was going to become an "it" instead of a person. I was scared. I let Doris know that my return to work had to be postponed, she made sure she kept close tabs on me.

Mary and I were going to go out to celebrate her birthday together since no one else was doing anything for her. We didn't get to do it however because my surgery was the following day. I told her we would do something before she went home for the holidays, but I was too sick. I apologized to her. Mary also noticed that I was becoming more depressed, which was dangerous because of surgery. I was because I had to hurry up and take my finals and find a place to stay because the dorms would be closed since my original plans had to be cancelled. The idea of recuperating from surgery over Christmas break instead of going to Ottumwa to see friends was not my idea of fun. I originally was going to stay with friends in Ottumwa and try to see some other friends that I hadn't seen since I left.

Mary always worried about me after we became friends. When I found out I was going to have surgery the first time, Mary wanted to be there for me. I still wasn't sure of her and said no when I really wanted to say yes. But I enjoyed every time Mary came to see me. I felt sorry for Mary the night her roommate insisted on coming with her to see me; both of us had problems with that. I even enjoyed her when she came to visit me on Christmas Eve at the hotel, but I felt sorry for her when she found out I was spending Christmas alone. If Mary had told me she wouldn't be included in the family activities, I would have let her come back to spend the day with me.

The place where I was going to stay had steps so that was out. Then the doctors told me NO traveling. Mary invited me to come to Davenport with her so I wouldn't have to spend Christmas alone. I told her thank you but I wasn't allowed to travel and I really didn't know her mother yet. I found out later there was steps at her house too. She had blown her stack when I stayed in the dorm alone over Thanksgiving. This was just too much for the old Buttinsky. She was an inactive Licensed Practical Nurse.

Remember I said she was naive. Just before Christmas Mary had gotten a check from Social Security for six months. She just stared at the check. She called me and asked if she could come down to my room. I told her of course she could. She came in and handed me her check and asked me several times if it was real. It took some strong talking to her to convince her it was indeed real, that it was for her, and she could indeed cash it. She made one mistake by calling her mother and telling her about the check; the next day her mother picked her up early, they went to Davenport and it was all spent in one day. I felt sorry for Mary because she did not get very much of it for herself.

My second Christmas vacation after getting out of a home full of abuse was spent in a hotel room. I assured Mary I would be okay at the Iowa House. I would have company, I could work on my crafts and catch up on my reading. However I was so sick that I did not do any crafts or reading.

Both Mary and Marie saw me just before Christmas and they were both very upset when they found out I was spending Christmas alone. I assured both of them I would be alright. I also told them I would be bad company for anyone. We were all VERY disappointed though at the meal that was delivered to me by MEALS ON WHEELS. It definitely did not fit a bland diet and I got very sick from it.

Mary told me she would be back but I told her not to worry, so much. Between Christmas and New Years, Marie and her daughter came back up. My daily meal had just been delivered when they got there because I was unable to get hold of anyone at the office. When Marie looked at it, she told me she was going to take it to feed to her animals and she would try to find something more suitable for me. Marie asked me what I had been able to keep down; when I said nothing she became very concerned because I was four weeks post-op. Again she was being a mother hen. I understood why though because she had been there the whole time when things was rough at Indian Hills.

A few days later Rebecca and Ann came up and we had a belated Christmas. Rebecca had seen me just before I went home from the hospital; noone was happy that they let me out when I wasn't able to keep anything down and had severe diarrhea. Both Rebecca and Ann were Registered

91

Nurses and neither was happy that I still couldn't eat. I bundled up so that I could go out with them for a while, we went out to eat. We made it back to the hotel before I got sick and had to change clothes. Afterwards Rebecca and I played cards while Ann took a nap, then they went home. Mary called that night to see how I was doing, and like everyone else, she worried about my progress. She told me that she would be up the next day, I was glad because I needed some things. I told her not to worry about me so much, but she DID anyway.

Mary would come even if I told her not to because of the whether. I had promised to call if I needed help but didn't because I resented having to impose on people. New Years Eve Mary came up to see me. I asked her if she would do my laundry, she told me that was one of the reasons she came. After doing my laundry, Mary stopped to get us some hamburgers and a shake for each of us, halfway through mine I got sick and had to change clothes again. Mary asked me how long that had been going on; when I told her since surgery, she started worrying even more. We both talked for awhile before she went home. Mary wanted to come back one more time before we moved back to the dorm, but I told her to try to have some fun before school started, I didn't know at the time how bad things were at home for her. I assured her that I could go a week without help. She really didn't understand I hated bothering people and I wanted to be independent. It was bad enough to be in a wheelchair, I had not really accepted being dependent on a wheelchair yet since I had been walking everywhere since the age of five.

I would describe Fall Semester with Mary as being very interesting and challenging at times. I learned how to understand and ignore a Buttinsky. The one thing I noticed with Mary was I could talk to her. Really talk and she seemed to understand where I was coming from. Her major fault was at first she was continually trying solutions for me. She was/is a caring, helping person. She was/is so naive that she actually thought that all people were genuinely caring.

Like I said, I could talk to Mary. She'd come down to my room and we'd talk for hours. She would give suggestions which I didn't always listen to. Mary noticed EVERYTHING, especially my moods. She would get me talking about my past and I would soon be sad and scared. She could get me to laugh. When my bleeding was increasing, I became more depressed but Mary was able to get me to talk it out.

SPRING SEMESTER

As I went into postoperative depression, Mary recognized the symptoms. I was trying to accomplish too much by going back to work, classes, my dealing with my family in Ottumwa and my health. Mary and I ate breakfast and supper together. She'd come over for study breaks and we would talk. Mary asked me about what happened to me throughout my life. I told her I couldn't talk about it and it was necessary for me to keep everything inside. I would not let go of my emotions and this made Mary mad; she finally let me go. Boy did she get me to open up.

Mary got it in her head that I needed to cry. She was NUTS. I didn't cry. It took her about two weeks or so before she had me crying. For awhile all she had to do was say, "cry Debbie, you need to cry." I would start crying. Then I decided I wasn't going to cry anymore. Mary didn't like that. She'd tell me to cry, if I didn't cry she was going to hit me on the count of three, but she wouldn't hit me because she knew that would cause problems for/with me. I would cry. It was like I couldn't turn off her faucet. I finally could cry on my own without her help. Then Mary decided I needed to wear a nightgown. After being in a fire and because of the past abuse in my life, I would wear my clothes to bed and this would aggravate people to no end, but it was easier for me to walk when I got up during the night to go to the bathroom. She also decided that I needed to sleep under the covers. She literally stripped me, tossed me a nightgown, and threw me in bed; she promised to help me get dressed if there ever was another fire. Mary was stronger when we lived in the dorms than she is now. She talked in her monotone voice and I would fall asleep. For awhile I slept in a gown or T-shirt to shut her up.

Lola was suppose to take me to Ottumwa for a play. Mary was in Davenport sick but she told me to call her if something happened to Lola. I knew in reality that Mary needed to take care of herself but I called Mary at the prearranged time knowing she couldn't get me to the play because the whether was bad from an ice storm. I told Mary not to try driving because it was bad because I couldn't even get to class or work that day. However the next day Mary drove to Iowa City against everyone's advice, picked me up and drove to Ottumwa to see Marie. I finally started to trust her. Marie was in Drakesville resting and Mary wouldn't take no for an answer and drove to Drakesville after Marie's husband and I both told her NO. Although poor Marie had only had a few hours of sleep she told her husband she would see me. Marie and Mary knew how much it meant to me. I was now indebted to Mary.

Before, during, and after this time, Mary helped me whenever I had problems with people. If I couldn't make them understand how I felt or what I meant, Mary would talk to them for me. Sometimes people got so mad at us. Lola didn't like me getting so involved with Mary; but the night I called Lola to take all of my pills out of my room because I was suicidal, she realized how much Mary did for me and cared for me. That night Lola found out how serious I was about committing suicide and it was MARY who got help for me.

Diane and Ron got upset with me for talking to Mary about my problems. But at least I didn't see her as an authority figure. And in the end, it was because of Mary that I finally got help. Mary worked with Jim, after talking to Jim one day Mary came to my room crying because she had told him about a confidential conversation we had the night before. She was afraid I would throw her out of my room and never talk to her again. It took me a long time to convince her I wasn't mad at her and I definitely would not throw her out. In fact I felt more secure with her because I was in love with her. Later Mary told me she did this so I wouldn't get mad and quit being her friend. Poor Mary she really thought she had lost my friendship, but of course she didn't.

My boss, Doris, was finally able to understand what was going on with after having a talk with Mary that day. I remember getting SUPER mad at Mary one day when she told Doris about me coming to work sick. After the two of them talked, Doris called me in to her office to talk with her; Doris tried to get me to promise that I wouldn't take it out on Mary, but I wouldn't promise. I wanted to kill her because she had portrayed my trust. Mary was in line for supper when I got home, when I didn't join her, she knew I was mad. She got out of line and we talked about it, soon we were both back in line but we didn't talk much during supper.

As we were coming out of the dining area, Doris walked in to see if everything was okay. I told them to enjoy their talk and went to my room. Shortly thereafter, they were both at my door to make sure I was okay because neither of them had ever seen me that mad. I told them yes and we all talked for awhile. Doris told me she wanted me to feel that I could tell her if I wasn't feeling well because she could sense it every since I came back from surgery.

Mary tried to get our advisors concerned about my depression but she felt they humored her instead. She told me I was suicidal. I asked her how she knew; she told me she recognized the signs. She tried to get me to talk to someone. I couldn't. I didn't want to. She told me how she had gone through the "suicide revolving door." I told her about some of the abuse and told her she didn't know what I was going through; another BIG MISTAKE. We went to lunch.

The next weekend Mary went to Davenport, every pay day she had to go home so her mom could have all of her money. I knew what Mary was going through and felt really sorry for her. Mary was like myself, she wasn't wanted for herself as a person, she was only wanted for her money. Not a nice feeling.

I would be alone for two days and have the chance to try suicide if I really wanted to. I took the pills. I got sick as a dog but I didn't die. When Mary came back she knew something happened. I finally confirmed her suspicions. She talked to me like an old mother hen. She really had tried suicide several times and failed. She didn't let me out of her sight that night. Again she went to people and tried to get them to commit me. Nobody would listen to her. It was shortly after this period that Mary and I became closer in our relationship.

Still I was depressed. I was having even more trouble working and concentrating on studying. One evening when Mary and a son of one of her friends was visiting in my room, she noticed my eyes from the corner of her eyes and then she saw me take something out of one of my drawers. I had started to leave with my heart pills and a coke. She ran to the door and told her friend to leave, I felt I was taking her away from her friends when we started hanging out together more. Then Mary blocked the door and demanded to know the answer to her question, "Where do you think you're going?"

I told her "away."

"Not until you give me the pills!" Did she have some kind of nerve or what. I wanted to tell her get lost. By that time I was scared because she had a firm hold on my chair and had it tilted back. SHE WOULD NOT RELEASE IT UNTIL I GAVE HER THE STUPID PILLS. Five minutes later she had the pills and we were both crying.

"You have forty-eight hours to tell somebody and get some help before I tell someone " Mary told me. We sat there quietly for quite a while. Finally Mary told me to talk. We talked for quite awhile. I knew she meant it. She stayed in my room until I fell asleep. Then she sat in the hallway the rest of the night in case I decided to go somewhere. I got up to go to the bathroom and she asked me where I thought I was going? I told her to the bathroom if it was alright with her. Use mine, Mary told me. The next morning I went to see Ron and Lola.

Mary and I talked a lot after that since I couldn't really get the appropriate help because it was getting toward the end of the semester. As the two of us got to know each other better, we worried about each other all the more. Mary became very sick and had to go home for two weeks but I called her everyday. She came to Iowa City twice during this time to get assignments and to see me. Mary asked me several times to go home for Easter with her and I finally agreed to go with her. Coming to get me was one of her trips to Iowa City. This was where I met Peg and Ed, one of Mary's sisters and brother in-law. I made them uneasy with my eating and there were problems every since.

I was going to take a course for the summer to have a place to live. At this time the dorm was the only place I had to live. But after my second serious suicide attempt, we both knew I wouldn't make it without getting help. She refused to let me stay in an empty dorm all summer and go to work. Mary told me I didn't have to take a class just to have somewhere to live. At the end of the semester I agreed to go to Davenport with her. Just to shut Mary up! I could HELP her mother with expenses for my keep. Her mother and their boarder agreed.

Mary thought that the relationship that had developed between us was only because of the role playing to defuse the abuse that happened to me most of my life. However it was much more serious than that. She was so naive that she didn't realize that we had something more than role playing. Mary did know however that she enjoyed the time we spent together. When I told her we were having a serious relationship, she didn't believe it. I told her it was true.

Mary's reaction to this news was, "I have to have a drink!" Poor Mary did not know what to think or say. We talked and I attempted to explain to her what was happening. At first she had a lot of trouble understanding it, but now we are living together and are very happy. Our relationship has caused problems for some while others have accepted it finally, but either way we are happy and we love each other very much.

Things was, are and always will be rough for us, but we have, can and will survive what ever comes our way. We have both gotten stronger as a couple. Mary's mom, Dottie was very mad and hurt when I told her about the two of us. She still has trouble accepting it when Mary doesn't get invited to family events. Mary finally told her she wouldn't go anywhere that I'm not invited, this makes things hard for everyone. But Mary knows I'm there for her.

CHAPTER 17: SUMMER OF HELL

After Mary had convinced me that I wouldn't be hurt by anyone, I went home with her. But it wasn't soon before our summer of hell started. After I told Dottie about us she sterilized everything after one of us used anything because she thought I had AIDS and everyone was going to catch it from me. I didn't/don't have AIDS so there was no way anyone could get it from me.

We started moving our things to Davenport the last week of April but we did not start staying there full time until May 5. Mary thought we would be staying in one of the rooms upstairs but instead we were moved into the basement. Each day we would take things from either Mary's room or my room to Davenport after classes and work. What we didn't know until the middle of the week, Dottie was going through everything while we were gone the next day, but she especially went through my things. How we found this out was one night when Mary and I went down to play cards half of my clothes were hanging separately from the rest of our clothes; Mary asked her mother why and she told us she wanted them, to keep hell from breaking out, I gave them to her.

At least twice a week, Dottie would go outside and look in the windows to see what we were doing. Mary and I would sleep in depending on what we had to do that day or if it was the weekend. Another thing that Dottie was looking for was if we were having sex. We got tired of her games and covered the windows so she couldn't see in, this made her very mad. One night we came home thinking our pop would be cold in my little refrigerator, but instead we found both our refrigerator and fan

UNPLUGGED. After getting un mad we fixed them so Dottie couldn't do that again; I mean we were paying the bills so what was her problem anyway.

Between the two of us we were only suppose to have to give her mother, Dottie, three hundred and fifty dollars a month; but between our Social Security, In home health services, and our food stamps it ended up costing us over a thousand dollars a month, which was a big difference in my opinion. When ever Dottie needed money and neither of us had any, Mary was asked what did she, meaning me, do with her money; which was really none of her business.

During the three months we were there, I saw ELEVEN doctors and therapists. The eleven included a medical doctor, chiropractor, dentist, psychiatrist and therapist, neurologist, speech therapist, occupational therapist, physical therapist, and I can't remember the other two but you get the general idea. I had some kind of an appointment every day. Which upset Dottie very much.

The chiropractor, Dr. C, was able to help me get stable enough so I could walk halfway around the track, which was behind the house, I actually even made it completely around the track a few times. Dr. C was also able to convince me that all men weren't mean. I felt sorry for him because he was also Dottie's Bishop at the time and when Dottie found out about Mary and I, she went to him for advice. The two of us talked about the situation, and according to the rules of the Mormon Church, I should have been kicked out; but because Mary was Dottie's daughter, I could stay. However, if I didn't convert to the Mormon religion within a year, which I didn't, Dottie could refuse to let me stay at the house.

All that summer and the next year, Dottie tried to convert me and when she was unsuccessful in doing so, she kept asking Mary when she was going to drop me as a friend. Contrary to what people thought, Mary was happy when we were together. The two of us were a team and we would always take care of each other. Needless to say I never converted my baptism to the Mormon church.

The dentist, Dr. J, pulled my upper teeth and made some dentures for me. This was no easy task due to my cerebral palsy.

The medical doctor, JJ, was able to take me off most of the medicine that I was on; while the neurologists Dr. R was able to confirm that I indeed was having seizures. The seizures are borderline between migraine headaches and Epilepsy, which is common for cp patients to have.

Dr. H and Anna was able to get me stable psychologically and was able to refer and transfer me to Mental Health in Iowa City. The other therapists were able to do maintenance therapy with me in hopes of postponing my going downhill mentally so fast.

Toward the end of May, I felt that Mary and I should tell Dottie about our relationship. We had started doing sexual activities through our role playing of the abuse I went through, but Mary did not realize that it was more than that until I told her otherwise. Once Dottie had time to come to terms with it, she looked at me and then at Mary, whom she proceeded to tell her daughter that she was more intelligent than that. Still today, I am trying to figure out what intelligence has to do with sex. Dottie now had three strikes against me. First, I am lower class, second, I am disabled and three I am gay. Every time Mary gets sick or diagnosed with a new problem, her family thinks she has gotten AIDS from me and that is why she is sick. However, I can't give her AIDS because I don't have it.

Later that summer there was a family reunion and Mary introduced me as her new sister which didn't go over with anyone. By this time Dottie had a chance to tell EVERYONE about Mary and I. Everyone told Mary not to bring me with her if she came to visit, this hurt Mary very much. Jo, Pat, and Peg, Mary's sisters, told us that their husbands did not want me a foot near their house, but Pat let me in when Mary and Dottie went to visit. Junior and Don, her brothers made/makes sure they tell AIDS jokes whenever I'm around.

Halfway through the summer we went to Oklahoma to see Pat, one of Mary's sister, and her family. While there Mary and I needed to get away for awhile so we went to see the Mount Scott area but we got lost along the way. When we got back Jim, Pat's husband, tore into us for being late getting back. Mary told him we got lost and wasn't close to a phone to call and say we would be late. While we were gone all hell broke loose and Dottie got into a fight with Pat. Dottie wanted to leave right then and there but because Mary and I hadn't had any rest, Mary told her she had to wait until morning. We left the next day but Dottie refused to help Mary drive home.

Once home all hell broke loose. We had new rules to follow and if we didn't Dottie locked us out. If Dottie had something she wanted to do or have done, we better not have an appointment. On Thursdays when we went to Iowa City to work at the Free Medical Clinic, we had to come back to Davenport instead of staying in a hotel like we had been. If we were at Sue's, Mary had to tell her mother when we would be home and what we would be doing. It was like living in prison but instead we were both dealing with abuse.

One day Mary was super late coming home from an appointment and I got worried. Dottie was mad at me for not letting her go through my purse or Mary's bill fold and she got even madder when I called Sue, one of our friends, to see if I could come over until Mary got home. Luckily Mary was there and I asked her to come get me out of the house for awhile, she could tell something was wrong and told me to get ready and she was on her way. When she got there Dottie started tearing into her, when I tried to defend Mary, Dottie told me to SHUT UP and she came very close to hitting me that day. Needless to say we left and didn't come back until Dottie was asleep, or so we thought. Once in the house we were bawled out again. If we had somewhere in Iowa City to go to, I think we would have left that night.

In July I got notice that I had been accepted for housing assistance. Mary kept going back and forth on whether she wanted an apartment or live in the dorm. Towards the end of the month we finally decided that we would get an apartment. We told Dottie she wouldn't be getting rent from me in August because we would have to pay rent, a deposit, get the utilities hooked up and pay one of our University bills so we could get our funding for school. Believe me, she didn't like it but accepted it because she knew she would get most of Mary's money. Time was running out and we still hadn't looked for an apartment yet and that worried me. One day Mary told Dottie we were going to go get an apartment that day, I gave her a look of disbelief, but we did get one that day.About this same time Dottie told me I wasn't coming back to school with Mary and I had to stay in Davenport so she could have my money. This was a shock to me because Mary hadn't told me I wouldn't be returning to school. I was so mad and upset I wouldn't even talk to her. Finally, I asked Mary why she hadn't told me she was leaving me in Davenport while she went to school. She asked me what I meant; I told her Dottie said I was staying with her so she could have my money each month. After Mary got out of shock she assured me that we were both coming back to school, then she made sure Dottie understood that too.

I met a lot of Mary's friends that summer, and Mary got to meet a lot of my friends too. We didn't get the chance to have many fn and relaxing activities, but what we did do we enjoyed. The two of us even went to Chicago and Ottumwa for a couple of days.

Most of the summer when we weren't at appointments or doing things with/for Dottie we were at Sue's. Sue was housebound and needed someone to stay with her while her son went to class, work, or out for some fun. We had a lot of fun at times when we were at Sue's house. After having two of her friends reject her because of me Mary got brave and asked Sue what she would say or do if she found out we were having a relationship. Sue told us that she had no problems with it, then she told us that she had already figured it out. The reason we decided to tell her was that she wanted us to stay with her for a few days while her son was out of town.

I would tell Mary to go fly a kite where the sun don't shine; Mary was SO NAIVE that she didn't know what it meant. One day she asked Sue if s he knew what it meant. Of course Sue and I started laughing and Sue told her yes. Mary then asked her what it meant and Sue explained it to her. Mary was shocked because she didn't think I knew what it meant. Mary forgot that I knew/know "street" language so we both sat there trying to explain to Mary what certain phrases meant, however she still doesn't understand them.

I think that it would be fair to say that we were both glad when it was time to come back to Iowa City. At least we could live more freely and not be under her mother's rules, or so we thought. For every cent we spent on the apartment we had to spend on her mother or the house. Once everything was taken care of Dottie strongly told me that I was responsible for the bills in Iowa City and Mary had to pay the bills in Davenport. To this day we do not know what Dottie spent her money on.

Dottie knew that I had some credit cards so if she wanted something and couldn't get it herself, she would tell Mary to get it on the credit cards for her; because I didn't want Mary to get hurt, I usually allowed it. If Dottie called needing money and we didn't have it, I was sent to borrow it if possible. Like I said, I didn't want Mary hurt or mad at me, so I would do it. I would get flustered about this a lot, but I needed to protect Mary.

CHAPTER 18: OUR FIRST APARTMENT

No one knew that we had secretly taken our marriage vows between each other before we went to Davenport for the summer, so the apartment would be our first home together. Yes things would be hectic at times but all couples had a few rough times, that's what relationships were/are all about; getting through the rough times as well as the good times. We would have to fight what people thought or felt about us, but as many of our friends told and still tell us, as long as we are happy, nothing else really matters.

We were able to find an apartment in one day, the number we called usually didn't rent to students, but because we were non traditional students they thought it would be okay. The apartment was part of a duplex, on ground level so I could get my electric wheelchair in and out without very many problems. We were told that the apartment would be cleaned when we moved into it two weeks later, but it wasn't. When I wasn't at work, or we weren't in Davenport, we were cleaning. An example of how dirty the place was is it took EIGHT buckets of soap and water to clean the refrigerator and almost that many to clean the stove.

When I called Marie and told her our new address and about our apartment, she asked if we had very many pots and things; of course we really didn't because we lived in the dorm the previous year. Once Marie heard about the apartment, she went through her things at home and went to an auction to get things for our new home. When Marie had gathered up a car load, she called and told us she was on her way up. After we helped her unload the car, we took her out to eat, on the way home she told us she had one stop to make. We told her okay, I should have known it would be the grocery store. Needless to say, we didn't need very much for awhile. When she left, I thank her and asked her what we owed her, she looked at me and told me not to be ridiculous because I didn't owe her anything; she just wanted me to be happy and healthy. I was happy but healthy would always be a problem.

One advantage of having our apartment was that Mary didn't have to walk up and down Clinton Street looking for me if my wheelchair broke down; that happened several times while we were in the dorm. I would go out to get something and either my chair would run out of power, or a couple of times my chair caught fire on me. I was glad when that didn't happen anymore. Also, it was a nice quiet neighborhood and we didn't have to worry about some one setting off the fire alarm for fun.

At first, it seemed that Mary didn't like the idea of an apartment, it was a change from the original plans of living in the dorm. However, it turned out that the apartment was the right choice. Mid September Mary had to drop the semester because Dottie was having surgery. I advised Doris and my teachers that I would be gone for a few days so that I could be with Mary. Once Dottie got home, I was coming back and Mary was going to take care of her mother; again Dottie changed the plans on us.

The day of Dottie's surgery was hard on Mary because her brothers and sisters, Mo and Marty, a niece and nephew, were at the hospital but they didn't sit with Mary because I was there. Later when Mary and I were going down the hall to see Dottie, Junior and Don started telling aids jokes as we went by. I told Mary to ignore them and lets go see her mother. Mary was upset and crying when she came out of the room, I was trying to console Mary when her brothers and sisters told her to grow up. I wanted to kill them, she needed support not ridicule. After Mo and Marty saw their grandmother they came to the waiting room to check on Mary, I started to back away but they told me it wasn't necessary. We told M0 to tell everyone we would buy supper, of course everyone but Mo had plans; Marty said he would but he had to go to work and we understood that. Mo went and told everybody goodbye and came back to where we were, she told us if it was alright, she'd join us. I told her of course it was alright. That night was when Mo and Marty started to accept me a little bit.

Mary was unable to be two places at once at times, so she asked Dora, a friend to be my personal care attendant, that lasted for about two months. When we were out taking my walk one day, Dora wanted to stop at the neighborhood bar for a drink. I was going to order a coke but Dora told me she had ordered me a screwdriver and I WAS going to drink it. I had taken a tranquilizer before she came because we had a house full of company. Dora had brought her three teenaged kids, and Glenda, another friend, brought all of her kids with her. I came home swinging my cane in the air and feeling no pain. While Mary was explaining to Glenda and Dora why I couldn't drink, the phone rang, it was Harley telling me my grandmother had just died. I was drunk, my grandmother died and I had just found out that I was having another surgery two days after Christmas, not a good day.

Friends were trying to get us to make their holidays for them, but we had all we could handle for ourselves. Dottie was upset that Mary would not be home for all of the holiday break. Two days after I came home from surgery Mary had to go bring her mother to Iowa City for an appointment. While she was gone there were several people coming to do things at the apartment. I was sitting there and noticed that the rugs needed vacuumed — you guessed it, I got the sweeper out and vacuumed them; halfway through the job who should come in but Mary. Yes, I got bawled out for doing it but I reminded her how particular her mother was.

Glenda came over to go with Mary, because I wasn't suppose to ride yet, to help Mary drive home, I was getting house bound so I talked Mary into letting me ride with her. She finally agreed so she knew I wouldn't do anymore housework. I took a pillow to hold over my stomach or put behind my back in case I got sore. Dottie suggested we stayed all night but we both told her NO! Besides Glenda needed to get home to her family. On our way home, we stopped at Rudy's and brought supper home.

Halfway in the semester Mary came home through a friend, Tricia, without the car. To show you how dumb I was I asked where the car was before asking Mary if she was alright; if I had just looked, I would have noticed that Mary was badly shook up. Some one had ran a stop light and hit her and totaled the car. Tricia took her back and forth to classes until Mary arranged to ride Bionic Bus. I really felt sorry for Mary when she called Dottie and told her about the accident; instead of mother being sympathetic and supportive, she criticized Mary for several days. Dottie was more worried about how she would get Mary's money than she was about if Mary was alright. I was really upset with Dottie for her lack of understanding and support.

Later that spring, Dottie and Aunt Ruth came up to visit. We had been getting a lot of free stuff from one of the companies we ordered from so we offered it to them. BIG MISTAKE, it was like two jealous children fighting over the stuff. Then we took the two of them out to eat, again they acted like two jealous children afraid that one was going to get more to eat or spend more than the other.

I tried to be Mary's note transcriber for her since I wasn't going to school that spring semester. Mary would get frustrated with me because I couldn't keep up, believe me I was honestly trying; but with a occupational therapist and nurse coming in, recuperating from surgery, and trying to keep the house and have warm meals for her, it was hard at times. It didn't help that I was too slow or when we had a car we had to go to Davenport once or twice a week.

At the end of the semester Dottie offered to arrange for someone to bring us home for the summer. Neither of us really wanted to lose the apartment and both of us was going to take two classes to make up for the semester that we missed. Again, Dottie was unhappy with us, but the two of us had our space and we were relatively happy.

When there was a break between semesters, or a holiday, or if we were sick and had to sit the semester out, we didn't have to worry about each other, especially the one that would have been stuck in Davenport, because we had our OWN place. Our first home together as a couple, and we could live as a couple without anyone butting in to our business. Also, we didn't have Dottie spying on us and telling us what to do, that was worth a lot to us.

During breaks we could do whatever we wanted, eat and drink what we wanted and not have to worry about other people. I finally felt free and I was starting to see a happier and more relaxed Mary. Mental health told us that I was the one keeping Mary alive, maybe so, but we were both free from abuse and neglect from our families.

One of Mary's Aunts died that year so I went to Davenport with her so I could "dog sit" while her and Dottie went to the funeral. The other reason I didn't go was that I wasn't allowed at family functions.

CHAPTER 19: REST OF THE TIME AT THE UNIVERSITY OF IOWA

Fall of 1990 would find us settled into our apartment totally. We were signed up for classes, some of them we took together. We had another car but we used the Bionic Bus to get back and forth to classes. Mary was my care attendant and I tried to help her with class notes.

Mary and I worked on building up our collections. Mary collects racoons and I collect owls. The symbolism of the racoon is his mask that he hides behind, because Mary has Borderline Personality Disorder, she hides behind a mask at times. An owl represents freedom and up until recently I felt like I had freedom.

One of our classes required us to do volunteer work, so we both volunteered at the University Hospital, but there was a problem when I had to start wearing a protective head helmet so I left there and went to work at Wild Bill's Coffee Shop, later Mary switched from the hospital to the Crisis Center. The coffee shop was originally opened by a disabled man that needed a job to help him stay out of an institution. For awhile Mary and I went to the auctions at Sharpless for the teacher who was in charge of the shop, but we got in trouble for buying too much so we stopped. My job at the shop was cleaning and organizing, but when I had to get down to clean under the tables, that was just too much and I had to quit. Mary stayed with the Crisis Center for ten years.

Mary decided to take Statistics, which is a hard course let alone having learning disabilities and taking this course, during her junior year. The class turned out to be the "class from hell" for her. She would leave the house between 7:30 and 9:00 am and often did not return until 7:00 at night. When I was on campus I would take lunch and supper to her just to get her to take a break. Mary was not satisfied with getting a C for the course, but it was a grade that was WELL earned.

Dottie was gone for the holidays that year so we went to Davenport to house sit and take care of the dogs. We also saw Sue a lot during that time.

I can't remember if I worked other than for Mary during spring semester, but I do remember that we saved enough money for the two of us to go to Branson, Missouri for a few days that summer. We were very tired when we got home but we had a lot of fun. Harley was coming to Iowa City for Cancer treatments, so he would stop by to see us once in awhile; I had seen him at the hospital one day when I was there having tests done and we started seeing each other in our perspective homes. He even brought us home grown canned goods.

Our Junior year, 91 - 92, was fairly busy with medical testing. Mary had to have a mole removed from her bottom, I went over to Student Health to see how things were going and Mary was coming out the door; I asked her how she was and what the doctors said, she told me then she tried to convince me that she was going to class. About the same time the bus pulled up and asked Mary if she was ready to go home, I was relieved to know that she was going home. I told her that I'd see her later.

I was being tested for thyroid problems; once it was decided I had Grave's Disease, the hospital treated it with radiation, I wasn't suppose to have another radiation treatment for SIX months, but six weeks later another radiation treatment was administered thus killing my thyroid. I now was placed on a thyroid hormone replacement for the rest of my life.

Later that year, Mary had to have a Sigmoid test done. I don't quite remember how and why, but I was left in Iowa City while she went to Davenport to have surgery. I do know that Dottie felt victorious over taking control again when it came to Mary. I called that evening to see how Mary was. Dottie rudely told me Mary was asleep, she was fine and she wasn't going to be woke up to talk to me. I firmly told Dottie to have Mary call me when she woke up; she did and she let me know what she had found out and I felt better when I heard Mary's voice.

Shortly after school was out my father passed away. Harley made me promise earlier that year that I would go to my father's funeral; I went but no one from the family really wanted me there. When Harley came, I asked him to put a rose in my father's hand, Mother and Paula said no. Harley came and told me where he put the rose, which my mother and sister threw in the fireplace, and we went in together to see father. Sharon and Nina had sat in a separate room with Mary and I, after seeing where I was sitting a few of the visitors came over to express their condolences with me. Afterwards I went back to the hotel to rest for the funeral the next day. Again, I was treated badly by my family, but I did what I had to do as a daughter. At the cemetery I noticed that the funeral director had retrieved the rose and buried it with my father, I was grateful for that.

Both of us took the summer off from school to relax a little. No we didn't go to Davenport for the summer, we stayed in our apartment on Second Avenue. Mary did more volunteering at the Crisis Center because a lot of the volunteers went home for the summer. I stayed home and tried to keep everything done up so Mary could rest whenever she was home.

One of the nieces, Dee, got married that summer. I was told that I wasn't invited so I could dog sit for Dottie. At the reception Mary was asked where I was, she told everybody that Dottie told us I wasn't to come. When we went back after Mary brought Dottie home, I was told then by Dee that I HAD been invited to the wedding. I told her it was okay and at least I got to come to the reception for awhile. The two of us had some fun before driving back to Iowa City.

Our senior year was even more hectic. I went to work at the Hospital School in the dietary department. Mary came over to help me get the files in order because no one had the time to do so. But once they hired someone, the new boss did not appreciate what we were doing, so Mary quit helping me. When I had time, I finished the project. Dr. Tutor was still there and one day we took the time to talk about me and my condition. I was starting to go downhill at this time. Dr. Tutor told me if it hadn't been for my family, I would never had been released from the care of Hospital School.

Mary was tested for sleep apnea; she was told that she definitely had it along with congestive heart disease. When it was time to start using the furnace that year, we started to get sick and we were both sick all winter. Mary was so sick that we stayed in Iowa City for the holidays that year. At the end of the furnace season, we found out that we had been in carbon monoxide poisoning all year, that explained why we were so sick.

Because we were so sick, Mary asked Jo to call Dottie more often; Jo did call more and she talked Dottie into moving to Florida in June. Needless to say, we were shocked because we were going to move to Davenport and live with Sue so Mary could check on her mother more often. Dottie didn't like that idea so she decided to take Jo up on her offer.

We decided not to attend our graduation ceremonies because neither of us had anyone that wanted to come to see us graduate. The two of us went to Ottumwa for a few days instead.

109

We went up on moving day to see Dottie off, but everyone treated Mary like dirt because I was with her. Even Mo ignored us that day. Mary was going to bring her stuff to Iowa City but it had all been given away.

Mary had arranged for Beth, a girl from Dottie's church, to stay at the house for a year to make sure that Dottie was going to stay in florida. Beth however turned out to be irresponsible and she wrecked the house. At the end of the year, Mary sold the house to her brother Don. Every once in awhile when Dottie is mad at us, she will throw all of this up in Mary's face.

We were finished with school so the two of us took some time just to relax and have fun. Dottie came back in 1994 for a visit. She and Mary sold the house to her brother, Don.

CHAPTER 19: SECOND AVENUE

I tried to find a job in the fall of 1994, I had the skills for everything that I applied for but once people realized that my wheelchair was part of me doing the job I was turned down. We took a class through Vocational Rehabilitation instructing us how to apply for a job but no one would hire me because of my disability. One day while visiting Harley he told me he always knew that I wouldn't get a job but at least I got the higher education and far away from my family's reach. Harley still kept us supplied with fresh produce and/or home canned goods.

Sharon was starting to have more health problems, so Mary and I tried to visit her more. Mary was even able to teach her how to crochet. We usually took a meal with us or we would go get one later during our visits with Sharon. One day Sharon asked us what we wanted to eat the next time we came down and we told her roast with all of the trimmings and even though she didn't like to cook a lot, Sharon fixed it for us. The meal was delicious.

Mary and I went to Oklahoma to drop off some craft items and other things that Mary wanted Pat to have. Because Mary was told that Pat mad and didn't want to see her, we were going to come home after resting the next day. I kept telling Mary that we should make sure that Pat found the stuff before leaving; Mary finally let me call Pat to find out. Pat's first question was "where are you?" I told her that Mary was told she didn't want to see us and we were calling from a gas station before we left town. Pat firmly told me to tell Mary that we were to get ourselves to her house RIGHT NOW!

I went back to the car and gave Mary Pat's orders. We went to the house and I was going to sit in the car while the two of them talked but Pat told me to come in too. After talking for awhile Pat asked us when we had to go back, Mary told her we didn't have to go back at any certain time so we stayed for a few days and had a lot of fun. The day before we left Jim called Pat and checked on her. He wasn't very happy at the time to find out that we were there so Mary and I started to leave while Pat was on the phone. Pat told him she had to go. Mary and I had gathered our stuff and was on our way out the door crying when Pat stopped us in our tracks; she told us that she told Jim it was okay for us to be there. I told Mary to stay and talk to Pat but I was going to the car, or so I thought, Pat stopped me in my tracks.

After Mary and I calmed down, we talked and stayed the night. We were having breakfast when Jim called the next day, he asked what happened then he told Mary over the phone that we were welcomed there anytime. Pat passed away in 1996 and we kept in touch with Jim until he passed away in 2003.

When Mary went down for Pat's funeral, Jim asked her where "Little Bits," his nickname for me, was. Mary told him that it was best that I wasn't there because of family, Jim kindly told her that he wished I was there instead of half of the people that was there. When I called the one time he told me that from now on when Mary came, I was to come too. Mary stayed at a hotel and her mother shared the room with her. I felt very sorry for Mary but knew that I couldn't physically be there for her because of family.

Mary continued volunteering at the Crisis Center and I eventually started volunteering; when the Crisis line became too much I took an extended leave of absence. During this time I had problems with my natural family and had to go to court. Although I was innocent, Mental Health encouraged me to plead guilty to avoid going to jail. Part of my sentence included community service hours so I volunteered at the Food Bank until I was let go due to a disagreement.

We made some trips to Florida to see her mother but we couldn't stay very long because Dottie was afraid she'd get in trouble. After getting in trouble with Jo several times, Dottie moved into the duplex next door to us. We soon found out that was a BIG MISTAKE but couldn't do anything about it. I ended up in the county home for six months, but I was ab le to come home and Mary and I have stayed together every since.

Somewhere between 1995 and 1998 Mary became my in home health aide again, but instead of going back to Visiting Nurses we tried Mercy Home Health care and this is where we first met Kay. Kay was our Registered Nurse who for a long time did not know that I could talk. I viewed Kay as an authority figure and I did not trust authority figures (I still don't totally trust them today.) My psychiatrist at the time told me that I had to let Kay know that I had tried to hang myself due to frustration, pain, and depression. I was starting to go downhill physically and I was having a lot of pain and the doctors could not find out why. Mary was talking to Sue, another volunteer at the crisis center, and she recommended that we tried her doctor. Only one problem, Sue's doctor was a cancer doctor. Dr. King saw me as a favor to Sue because some of the problems I was having could have been cancer. Luckily I was cancer free but the medical problems that were found would be with me the rest of my life.

In 1998, I left the home health program because I did not feel that I needed it. Kay and I had became friends. When Kay had her second neck surgery, I went to visit her once a week and this is where I met her husband, Joe, and her son Toby. Joe is a retired fireman and Toby was a student at the time; I met the rest of Kay's family later that year. Shortly after Kay's neck surgery, I had to have my gallbladder out. Because Mary didn't trust me, she would have me ask Kay if I could visit her while Mary either went to class or to work a shift at the crisis center. Kay usually said yes.

In 1999, my doctor convinced me to go to the hospital for a few days. However, it was bad timing for Mary because her mother was having surgery at the other hospital around the same time; needless to say, I wasn't there for Mary during her mother's surgery. I had planned on only being in the hospital for a few days, but health problems, including a heart problem, kept me there for twelve days. Mary was completely wore out by the time I came home and even more wore out when her mother came home six weeks later.

On January 17, 2000, Mary slipped on some ice and broke her back after going outside when the

Seats driver told us that Dottie had fallen and the ambulance was on the way. Mary kept telling the ambulance drivers and myself that she was okay, but we convinced her different. Kay and I was in the emergency room with Mary when she teasingly said she broke her back, the doctor came in at that time and told us that she did indeed break her back; but because she had not used her Medicare spend down yet, they sent her home.

Kay and Joe would bring groceries or meals to us as friends and because they did not want me out in my electric wheelchair in the dead of winter. They didn't realize that I needed to get out every so often because of my mental illness. Later Kay and Joe would become part of our care team and Toby would be the one to help us with computer problems. Mary and I felt like they were adopted family to us.

February 2001 found me going to an adult center during the day to help get me out among people. At first I enjoyed it but as the center got more people and I needed more help, it was time for me to move on. In my mind I knew that I was getting worse, but in my heart, I didn't want to accept it. AND THAT IS STILL TRUE TODAY!!

We help each other as much as possible but our health was making it necessary for us to start thinking about moving to a different safer place. One day, Patty, our local DHS worker told us about some new apartments coming up for the handicapped and elderly. One day Kay had seen one of the apartments and liked so she brought the two of us by to see them. We told her she could pick up an application, which she did while we were with her, and we filled it out. The first building was almost filled but a second building was being built so we waited for that building to open up.

In the meantime, one day while I was at camp Mary took Dottie by and showed her the complex and told her we might be moving there. What Mary didn't know was that Dottie wrote the number down and called the next day to have an application sent to her. Yes, Dottie moved into the first building before we got to move in. Kay helped us pack to move and we found people to help us move.

CHAPTER 20: SHANNON DRIVE

February 2002, we moved into our new home, our second home as a couple. It took a while to get things the way we wanted them but we were happy. I quit going to the adult center and the two of us adjusted to our new home. At the time I was in case management and Carla, a Social Worker from Ottumwa, who is also a long time friend, came for her annual visit. She seemed pleased with our new home. Mary and I would go out into the community room to play games, do puzzles, or just to visit with some of the other residents. Eventually however rumors were started about us and we were asked to stay in our apartment so that the other residents could enjoy the community room. We were hurt, but we did as we were asked. Now we play our games and do our crafts in our apartment.

In 2002, Mary lost her balance and fell in the bathroom; she hurt her hip and had to start using a

walker. Mary was hoping to get rid of the walker once her hip healed, but the chiropractor wanted her to use it and Mary fought it constantly, but she finally gave in and took it with her when she was going to be outside of the apartment.

December of this year brought us a lot of sad news. Mary had been having more and more health problems but we didn't know why. Two days before Christmas Mary was informed that she had MS and had suffered several TIA'S (mini strokes.) Needless to say, this was a shock for both of us. We now started taking life day to day.

January 1 - September 8, 2003

I had quit taking my vitamins for a while and got to the point where all I could do was pivot from one place to another. On the fifth of January, I received a call telling me that my mother was in a nursing home and not expected to live very long. Two days later I went to see her but I thought she was going to be around for a while. The two of us made peace and I called her everyday even though she didn't really know who I was. The one thing mom did remember was that I had been there and given her a rose. I was told she carried that rose everyday with her. Mom wanted to go home and I thought she meant back to the house, when in reality she was telling me she was ready to die.

I made it a point to call mom every day. On Friday of that week, mom mentioned that she hadn't talked to me, that was only because I was told I was no longer able to talk to her. That night she went to the hospital and died January 12th at 8:30 pm. I knew mom was in a better place but her death was a shock for me. Two days later I went to Ottumwa to bury my mother. I went to the funeral home the next day and greeted people that came to pay their respect to mom, but my sister never came. I was invited by the minister to come to the dinner at the church before the funeral. I was hesitant, but Mary, Kay, Joe, and I went, but my sister and nephew let me know that I was not welcomed there.

By March, I realized that I needed some help mentally. I tried a psychiatrist on my own, but that didn't work out so Carla arranged for me to see someone she knew and I have been seeing Dr. O every since. Also in March, Mary had a TIA and it damaged her left eye, we will soon find out if she will be able to get her sight back.

In April, we had three more deaths. Sharon's dad died the first part of the month but we were unable to be there for her. On Easter, Mary's Aunt Ruth died and the next day Jim, the brother-in-law from Oklahoma died. We were torn between two funerals, we were committed to stay in Iowa to get Dottie to her sister's funeral, but we wanted to be in Oklahoma because we were close to Jim.

Kay, Joe, Mary and I went to Kansas City and Ottumwa in May. We had a lot of fun. We went to a zoo and to Mary's Church Temple. Sharon was glad to see us, but she noticed that Mary was going downhill fast, she keeps us in her daily prayers.

June and July found me having more trouble with falling from my wheelchair and/or having accidents by hitting potholes. I went back on my vitamins and started doing better but it was too late. In the middle of July I was out in my wheelchair and lost control. Instead of going into four lanes of traffic I decided to try for the curb cut, but I hit the curb and fell forward with my wheel chair landing on top of me. I injured my elbow and we are uncertain what other damage I did yet.

Six weeks later, Mary slipped on some water in the kitchen. She broke three toes, sprained a knee, bruised her back and hit the back of her head. While she was in the hospital, the push for us going to a nursing home was started. At the ages of 49 and 57, this is not something one wants to hear. A week after she came home Carla, Patty and Kay was at our house urging us to start thinking about putting our names on some waiting lists. We agreed to do so put we told Carla and Patty that we wanted to pay off our bills and pay for our cremations before going into the nursing home. We will have to wait to see what life allows us to do.

Today, Mary and I still hurt and feel betrayed but we take each day one at a time. Frustrated and scared — YES, but we have each other and that is what really counts!!

CHAPTER 22: FIFTIETH BIRTHDAY PARTY

In January Mary and I were trying to figure out what to do special for my fiftieth birthday. The two of us were talking amongst ourselves and decided to have a party. A CELEBRATION OF LIFE is what we referred the party to. We planned it and really had fun doing it. In fact, we both looked forward to having the party. The reason we called it a celebration was because I was not suppose to live past thirty due to my cerebral palsy.

After deciding on a date, six days before my actual birthday, I got the disc out and made my own invitations. On the outside of the invitations it said: Great American Classic which I felt was appropriate. I had a lot of fun doing it but drove everyone crazy because I tried to do things too soon. Needless to say, the time went faster than what people thought it would. I knew within just a few days how I wanted the party to be. Mary got very frustrated with me because I kept doing everything and not letting her and th aide who was co-hosting do anything. Because Mary really didn't have a way to get out, I tried to do it all. But eventually, I think she forgave me.

We sent out several invitations and furnished all of the food for the event. I even invited my natural family, but no one came. One cousin tried to get here but had an accident close to her home. For food, we supplied the making for sandwiches, salads, chips, candy, cake, ice cream and drinks. On my actual birthday, there was a pizza party in the complex.

Jill, another resident who lives in the same building also had a birthday on the same as mine, so we had a double celebration. It was a lot of fun. Many of the residents, our friends, and some family on Mary's side came. I had told most people just their coming was enough and not to buy any presents, but many did not listen to me.

I had always wanted a picture of Mary and I together, when I received a stained glass picture frame, I finally got my wish; our cat, Muffin was even in the picture. We had a friend take a snap shot of us then I took it up and enlarged it so that the picture would fit the frame.

EPILOGUE

Elvis Presley summed up life fairly well in his song, MY WAY! Here are his words:

MY FRIEND, THE END IS NEAR SO I FACE THE
    FINAL BURDEN.
I DID IT ALL, I TOOK IT SLOW, BUT MOST OF ALL
    I DID IT MY WAY!

Yes, I have done it my way. It has been a long struggle, but the fighting will continue until the end. I have tried to make something with my life and that is what gives me the strength to write my story.

I came into this world severely handicapped, I will leave this world severely handicapped, but I am not biter about this fact. In fact, I feel that my handicap has given me a chance to learn things most people do not get the opportunity to learn ... mainly because I had to learn these things where most people do not have to learn them. The only regret in life that I have is that people always told me that I would be able to fulfill my dreams; when deep down, these same people knew that this was not true. My dreams included getting a degree in Library Science, then it was Social Work, and I ended up getting a degree in English. My idea of life is not waiting month to month for a government check as I do now, but to work and feel that it is worthwhile to live. Deep down I still feel I can do this, but in reality, I know that I will never be able to work for a living.

One of my pastimes is listening to music. I enjoy listening to the radio, records, CDs and/or cassettes. When I was younger music seemed to bother me for some reason, but now I really enjoy it. As I wrote this book, there were many songs that went through my mind. I have used some of these songs or titles to express some of my thoughts and feelings.

I was once asked how I viewed life since I was handicapped. I didn't have an answer then but I feel I could give an answer now. I view life on Earth as one with many trials and tribulations. Every day life has been a constant battle for me and I learned many lessons from life, such as adapting activities to meet my needs, that most people will never need to.

Well this is my life story up to today. I hope that you enjoyed reading it as much as I enjoyed writing it. Although the abuse was there, I think I was to show you the fight with my handicap was what I really had to endure more to survive. But there is one thing I must say: please don't feel sorry for me just because I'm a little different. It is through my being different that I have seen many things that you will never see. Of course, if you cannot see something, you will not understand it either.

I do want to say that each and every person has a handicap whether it is noticeable or not. That is why I am no longer ashamed of being handicapped. The change in today's society's attitude toward the handicapped has made it easier for these people come out of their corners of hiding; handicapped people can teach ALL of us about determination and courage. This is one of life's most valuable lessons. So please take time to learn it with me. Then I too can BE A PERSON!

About the Author

A woman in a wheelchair who has difficulty speaking, someone calls her retarded. She makes a phone call, someone else tells her she's drunk and hangs up. You feel outraged for her. She grins, smiling and says she is retarded. You're dumbfounded! Again she smiles and say, "I'm respectable, educated, tolerant, accepting, resourceful, determined, excited and dependable." She's teaching you patience. Another time, a miss do-gooder is making some suggestions about some adaptive equipment, she smiles and says, "I've had cerebral palsy for a few years now." I'm teaching you tolerance.

Jen has a story to tell. It's finished! She has struggled to live, to move, and even to speak. She has Cerebral Palsy, the "hell" disease as it effects every one of her limbs, muscles, nerves, and organs. As she fights, people along the way help teach her love, compassion and patience. She sees others with the disease lose their battle against it. She learns to fight discrimination and ignorance. She fights for her dignity and wins the respect of others. She continually overcomes physical and emotional abuse.

Jen has celebrated her fiftieth birthday, living twenty years longer than she was suppose to have lived. Self acceptance is not easily won but can be obtained.

www.ingramcontent.com/pod-product-compliance
Lightning Source LLC
Chambersburg PA
CBHW051422280526
45785CB00003B/1128